Herbal Remedies Starter Kit For Optimal Health & Vitality

Create Your Homemade Apothecary With Medicinal Herbs & Plants in 5 Steps or Less

Amber White Dawn

ISBN: 979-8-9872425-1-3 / Paperback

Cover Design by Amber White-dawn
E-book Interior Design by Amber White-dawn
Illustrations by Heoh Kim
Editing by Susan Johnson

Published in the United States of America

Have questions or need support on your herbal journey?

Come Join Our Herbal Family!

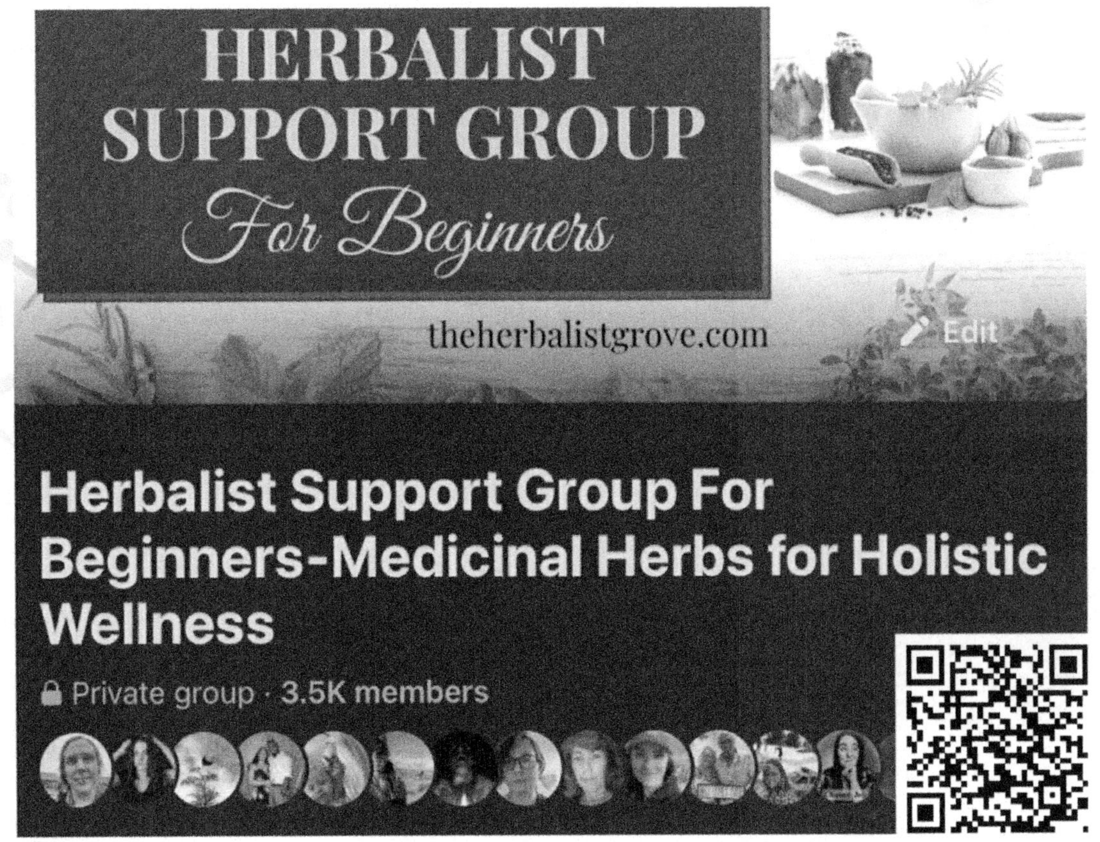

Connect with like-minded individuals in our private Facebook community!

GO TO Theherbalistgrove.com or

SCAN the QR code above to

JOIN NOW!

Dedication

To my mother, Susan. You have always believed in me and told me I could do anything I set my mind to accomplishing. You believed in me even when I didn't believe in myself. Your strength and dedication to being a phenomenal mother are an inspiration, and I love you more than words. I could not have written this book without you. Thank you for helping me edit, encouraging me to keep going, and pushing me to share my love of medicinal herbs and plants with the world!

Contents

Contents

Introduction

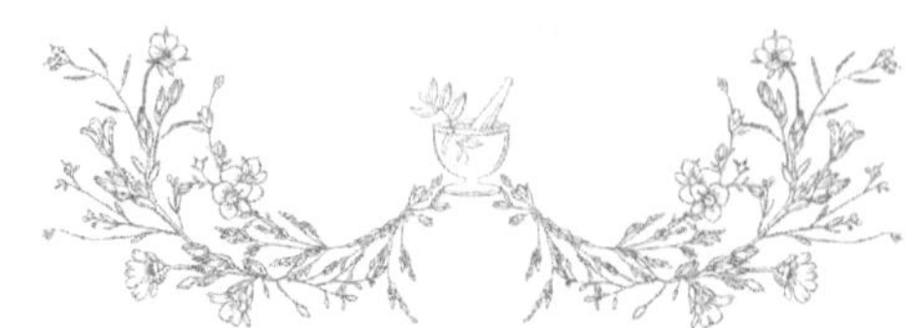

The alarm went off, and Jane got up feeling fabulous. She sat in bed and stretched her arms out to greet the day ahead before tiptoeing to the kitchen. She placed water on the stove and added a few herbs to brew tea. Looking at the water boiling in the pan, Jane smiled as she watched the green leaves moving around in the peace of the early morning. She switched off the stove, strained the tea, and silently sat with it. The hot liquid felt warm in her hands, and Jane took a sip.

As Jane enjoyed her lovely warm tea, she thought, *"Hmm, this is sheer bliss."* She was mindful of the liquid touching her lips and going down her throat. Warmth spread and engulfed her entire body. This daily ritual of tea meditation energized her to face the hectic day ahead.

After finishing her morning routine, Jane munched on the sandwiches she had made the previous night. The mint and lemon juice she had used to create a spread on the bread was tasty and satisfying. She knew the mint would help keep her acid reflux in check and allow her to be free of heartburn throughout the day.

Jane suffered from acidity, heartburn, and acid reflux. Her stomach got bloated and felt stiff as it filled with gas. No amount of antacids gave her relief, while prescribed antibiotics and medications only provided a temporary respite. She was eventually diagnosed with colitis as the internal walls of her intestines were bleeding.

At this point, Jane was looking for alternative care and came to see me. She was completely stressed and exhausted. Jane panicked and told me about her problem. I reassured her that she was validated in her discomfort, gave her an herbal massage with chamomile oil, and afterward asked if she had ever heard of herbology. Curious about it, Jane requested me to elaborate. I explained how herbal wellness programs help people enjoy optimal health and vitality. With my brief explanation, Jane continued to seek my support. I was glad to educate her about the wonders held inside of Mother Nature!

Together, we chalked out a meal plan and simple lifestyle changes essential for general wellness. Knowing Jane's acid reflux concern, I explained how acidity occurs and suggested eating small quantities at frequent intervals. Jane added fresh herbs to her diet and munched on fruits between meals. She avoided fried and gas-producing foods. She also received a monthly massage to help remove toxins and keep the energy flowing smoothly throughout her body. Jane felt refreshed, rejuvenated, and raring to go. Within six months, she felt upbeat about life as her heartburn slowly stopped, and the acidity was under control. No more belching or farting.

Jane is one of many people looking for a more natural way to approach wellness. Like Jane, you can also find relief from your common ailments and feel rejuvenated. The forthcoming chapters will reveal all the herbs and plants that will assist you on your journey toward optimal health and vitality. You will also discover remedies to make and keep on hand for future use.

Contrary to popular belief, medicinal herbs and plants are not only used by alternative practitioners. Herbal medicine is a precursor to modern pharmacology. About one-fourth of all prescription medicines come from herbs and other plants. The centuries' worth of herbal medications led many physicians and researchers to take a new look at traditional herbal remedies.

You do not need to run off to the doctor for common ailments, although you should always check with your doctor before consuming any supplement or herbal remedy. There are plenty of natural solutions available to produce at home or find in your local herbarium. Supplements and herbal concoctions are excellent alternatives to synthetic chemical compounds found in pharmaceuticals.

Herbalism can also help balance mental, emotional, physical, and spiritual distress. When we consume things in our minds, they can express themselves in the body. Conversely, when we absorb nutrients into our bodies, they can reflect in our minds. For example, emotional agitation and turmoil can often express themselves in an agitated and overwhelmed digestive system. An angry red mood may sometimes reflect a red hot, sore blister.

As we become more aware of ourselves, we also become more able to embody our inherent wisdom to nourish ourselves. Mother Nature has showered us with her bounties, and with the assistance of herbal remedies, optimal health and vitality await!

Herbal Remedies & The Modern World

There is a misconception that traditional medicine is a magic potion that can cure all illnesses. You may have probably read somewhere that such-and-such herb cures cancer. Though this may have been true in a specific instance, traditional medicine differs from modern (allopathic) medicine. There are numerous notable differences to look into on the subject!

The main difference is in the approaches to diagnosis and treatment. Modern medicine has tremendous advantages. Surgery has been a big help for people suffering from acute conditions or physical trauma. Let's not forget that many thousands of people live happier and longer lives due to modern medicine. Without our physicians and hospitals, who knows where the world would be? You may ask yourself why you should choose herbal remedies if modern medicine can cure all ills. This question is an excellent one to ask for several reasons.

Modern medicine looks at the symptoms and offers a cure. For example, a physician would suggest a pill if you have a headache. Your headache may disappear immediately but the pill does not necessarily address the root cause of the headaches. In traditional herbal medicine, the practitioner looks at the whole person holistically. You may find relief from your headache over some time while addressing the underlying cause.

Herbal medicine is a lifestyle choice, which can lead to a better, more wholesome life. You will discover a whole new and beautiful world with herbal solutions and begin to feel energetic and lively. You will live life with zest and enthusiasm. You will live passionately and love passionately. You may find that you never again have to encounter common ailments because you will be leading a healthy life – free of chemical-based pharmaceuticals. Opting for herbalism can give you relief from issues that may have been plaguing you for years.

An imbalance in your body causes illnesses. This imbalance exhibits itself in several ways.

For example, your stomach may ache because of acidity. Simply taking a pill for the issue may relieve you, but the problem will remain dormant and can reappear. With an herbal lifestyle, the root cause of the problem will be directly managed and addressed.

It would be best to look at all areas of your life that need balance. Do you have a nutritious diet? Are you getting enough good quality sleep? What do your exercise and movement routines look like daily? How do you manage stress? The comfort you have been searching for comes when you change your dietary habits to include herbs and plants. This lifestyle is only possible when you look at the root cause of your ailments on your journey toward optimal health and vitality.

What Are Herbs?

Now, let us talk about herbs! They are different from spices and are sometimes categorized as vegetables. Spices come from dried seeds, roots, barks, and fruits, whereas herbs are short leafy flowering plants with green, delicate, tender stems. They do not have branches, but their thin, soft stems may "branch" out with leaves. Throughout this book, you will see the terms herb, spice, and medicinal plants used interchangeably depending on the plant being covered.

Many herbs are available in nature. Gathering wild edibles is known as wildcrafting or, more commonly called, foraging. However, be careful! You should only wildcraft if you are 100% confident in your identification. Many field guides can assist you in identifying medicinal herbs and plants in the wild.

Herbs can surely provide your body with a variety of benefits. They add different tastes to food, and you can use them in your cooking to boost your immunity. They contain micronutrients like vitamins and minerals your body needs to grow strong and healthy. Some herbs commonly used to garnish foods also add fragrance to the home. A small pot of rosemary or mint can exude aroma and also works to keep food fresh.

Herbs are used not only in food but also for medicinal and spiritual use. For example, burning sage can keep the negativity away from your home and help you meditate in peace. Massaging your body once a month with herbal oils can strengthen your bones and allow free blood flow throughout your body. Massaging with essential oils not only works well for your body but also polishes your skin and gives it a shine. In this highly polluted world, herbs and their oils can help you enjoy optimum health and vitality.

Hundreds of herbs are used in food and medicines worldwide, and it can be advantageous to grow your own at home. You can quickly cultivate cilantro, clove, thyme, and dill on your window sill. They do not need much care and can be a great place to start your herbal experience. Imagine having an herb stand in your kitchen window where you can pluck a few leaves and garnish the food as you prepare it. It is fresh and aromatic as well as fuel for your health. Read on to discover what Mother Nature has bestowed on us to lead a remarkable life.

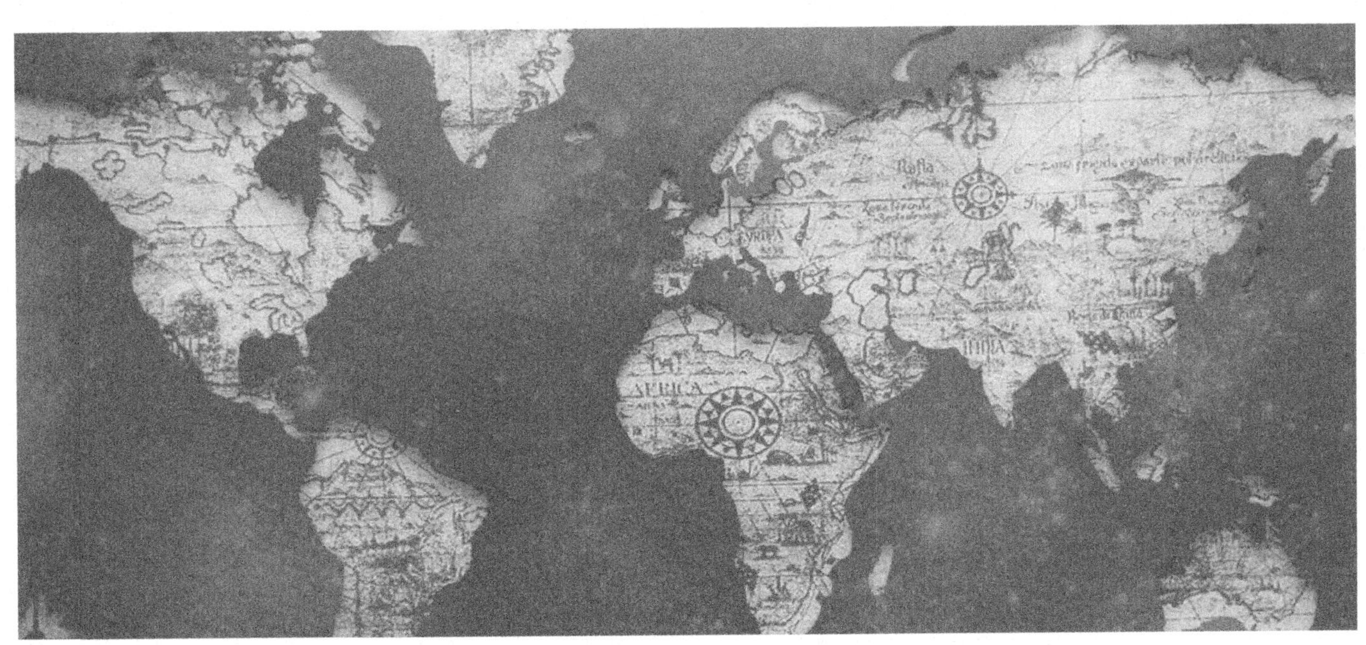

Chapter 1

The Magical World of Mother Nature's Medicinals

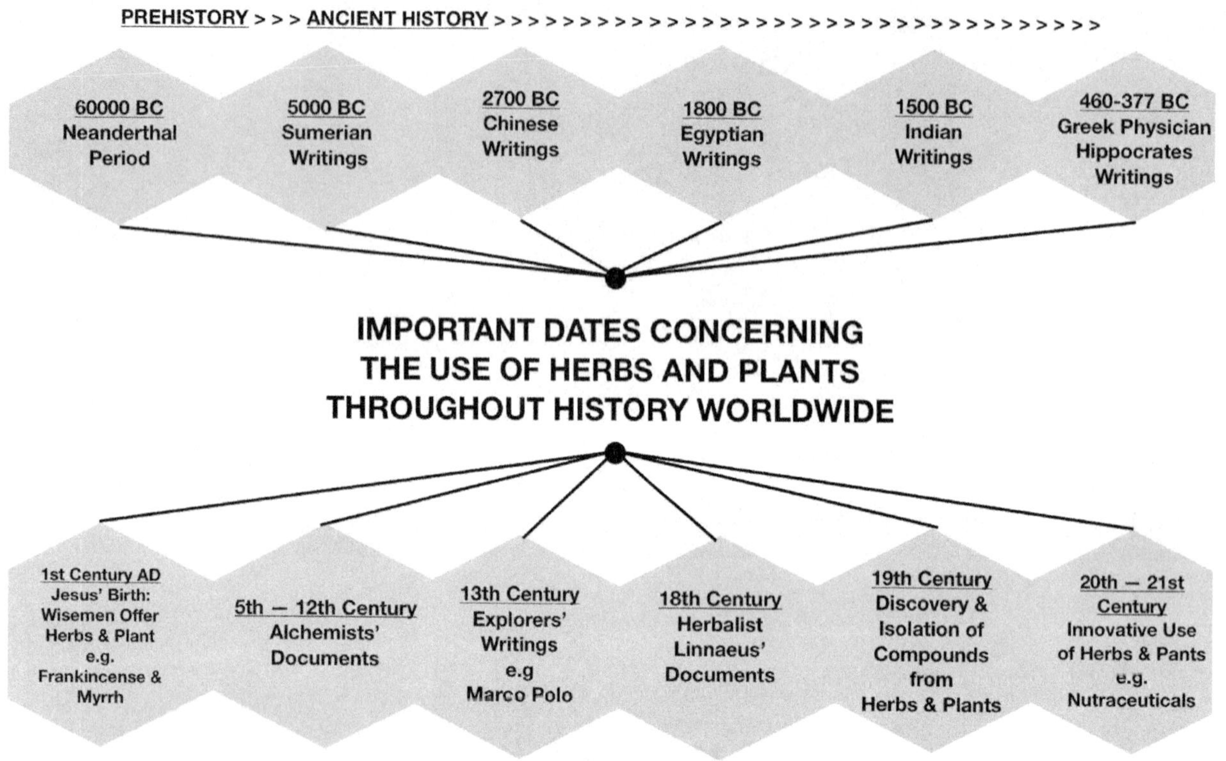

Prehistoric History

Herbalism is something that you will encounter in our modern world. However, herbalism is not a new phenomenon! Evidence shows that medicinal herbs and plants started as far back as the Paleolithic period. In 1960, archeologists discovered a neanderthal man in northern Iraq. This man was seen buried with eight different plant species. Such a finding is remarkable because some of those very plants are still used for their medicinal properties today.

Similarly, in 1991, archeologists found another prehistoric burial site on the border of Austria and Italy in the Ötztal Alps. Historians believe the neanderthal, known as *'Ötzi the iceman,'* lived between 3400 and 3100 BC. Found with medicinal herbs in his personal belongings, they think the iceman used them for the parasites found in his intestines.

Ancient History

Historians found the oldest written recording of herbal remedies in Nagpur, India, on a Sumerian clay tablet nearly 5000 years old. The evidence showed a dozen recipes for drug prescriptions harnessing the medicinal properties of between 200 and 250 different plant varieties. In the Sumerian civilization, the physicians formed a paste of several herbs to use on wounded soldiers during war times. Furthermore, records on cuneiform tablets in Mesopotamia date to around 2600 BC. During this time, many ancient civilizations started to take a more scientific approach to medicinal herbs and plants.

By 2700 BC, the Chinese began to look at herbs and plants scientifically. Around 2500 BC, the Chinese Emperor Shen Nung completed a book on roots and grasses called *'Pen T'Sao.'* The compilation consisted of 365 parts of dried medicinal herbs *(Petrovska, 2012)*, and many of the plants mentioned are still widely used worldwide.

Most Chinese medicines originate from plants and herbs, and the practice would become known as Traditional Chinese Medicine (TCM). Although TCM encompasses many other disciplines, such as acupuncture and massage therapy, herbal remedies are the foundation of this healing practice.

Around 1500 BC, recordings of herbal medicines were illustrated on walls and written on papyrus during the Old Kingdom of Egypt. One important document to note at this place was *'The Ebers Papyrus.'* These recordings contained over 800 prescriptions and references to over 700 plants utilized for medicinal properties *(Petrovska, 2012)*. Some of the plants mentioned in this document, including aloe vera, garlic, juniper, and onion, are still used today.

Herbal knowledge during this time is not limited to medicinal concerns. There is mention in Egyptian history that Queen Cleopatra used beetroot powder mixed with oil to make her lipstick. Also, orange peels were used as face powder and masks, while sweet berries were adorned as necklaces and bracelets to entice men. Biting the berries around the neck was a prelude (foreplay) to sex by the ancient tribes.

The rich history of India also shows significant applications of herbal approaches. Some historians date the record back to the early writings of Ayurveda, around 1500 BC *(Ravishankar, 2008)*. Many herbalists today are mindful of the value of Ayurvedic teachings. It is an ancient Indian medical treatment for illnesses that address the ailment and aids in general well-being. Furthermore, these teachings focus on balancing bodily systems with the help of diet, breathing exercises, and healing herbs. The practitioners of Ayurvedic medicine even consider the environment and weather conditions.

Siddha is one of the oldest medical practice forms in South India. Siddha is more or less like Ayurveda yet combines mysticism, spirituality, and herbalism. Siddha was popular from 2500 to 1700 BC during the Indus valley civilization. The rich knowledge from Indian history and Ayurvedic teachings is still noticeable in the modern era. Many Indian medicinal herbs and plants, such as pepper, nutmeg, and clove, are still used today.

Next, as we follow the timeline through ancient history, we come to the prominent *'Father of Medicine,'* Hippocrates. His writings date to around 460–377 BC, and he compiled between 200 and 300 different medicinal plants classified by their physiologic actions. For instance, some of these writings mention how garlic can be utilized for its healing action against parasites, while parsley, celery, sea onion, and asparagus aided as diuretics *(Hassan, 2015; Petrovska, 2012)*. Hippocrates founded the Hippocratic School of medicine and was famously quoted saying, *"Let food be thy medicine and medicine be thy food."* He was one of many Greek philosophers that indulged their curious minds with the magic of medicinal herbs and plants.

Aristotle, a student of Plato, is another famous Greek philosopher. With the help of his student Theophrastus, he collated medicinal herbs, studying the parts of which plants had medicinal qualities and their effects on human beings. Historians believe he compiled most of his work between 335 to 323 BC while in Athens *(Sallam, 2010)*. Inspired by the plants growing in Athens, Aristotle started the science of Botany and medicinal plants.

Medicinal Plants In Biblical Times

Applications of several herbal lifestyle methods have also been recorded in the Bible. Only five medicinal plants were mentioned by scholars directly in the Bible: fig, nard, hyssop, balm of gilead, and mandrake. However, evidence of the use of medicinal plants in Egypt and the surrounding areas dictates logic that their use as Biblical Medicinal plants is plausible *(Dafni & Barbara, 2019)*. Furthermore, we also see stories involving these plants, like that of the wise men's offering of frankincense and myrrh at the birth of Jesus. The Bible also notes that they covered Jesus in aloe and myrrh before being wrapped in linen cloth after his death.

Alchemists Documents & The Dark Ages

Hermes Trismegistus (c. 580–470 BC) was an infamous alchemist throughout the Middle Ages. He became so famous that alchemy is often called *"hermetic science."* Thought to be the medieval forerunner to modern chemistry, alchemy became crucial in developing the healing properties found in herbs and plants throughout medieval times.

People encountered countless deadly ailments during the first part of the Middle Ages. Because of this, the Middle Ages were also referred to as the Dark Ages. Whether it was malaria, tuberculosis, smallpox, diphtheria, measles, or leprosy, Europe was running scared. That is where medicinal herbs and plants came to the rescue.

In AD 77, the Greek physician Dioscorides made significant contributions and became known as the *'Father of Pharmacognosy.'* His writings, *'De Materia Medica,'* compiled over 900 drug recipes, of which 657 came from plants *(Hassan, 2015; Petrovska, 2012)*. His writings became the dominant documents in Europe for over 1,000 years and were translated into several languages.

During the Middle Ages, healing practices moved to the monasteries, where monks would cultivate herbs and plants to prescribe for ailments. Much of the monks' knowledge came from Dioscorides' documentation in *'De Materia Medica,'* the most widely referred to work in Europe between the 5th and 12th centuries. Galen (c. AD 130–200) became commonly referenced as well. Galen was a physician and pharmacist who influenced the development of various scientific disciplines and documented the use of plants as medicines, some of which were not mentioned in Dioscorides' documentation.

The *'Saxon Leechbook of Bald'* is England's oldest surviving herbal manuscript. Historians believe it was written around AD 900–950 by a *'team of compilers'* under the intellectual sponsorship of King Alfred *(Hajar, 2012; Scott Nokes, 2004)*. Prescribed herb baths became standard practice for a myriad of ailments. The book gives detailed accounts of crusaders bringing back all kinds of perfumes from the Middle East. The most prestigious of all was rosewater. The nobles would use it in perfume baths and display bowls of rosewater for guests to wash their hands after meals.

The Europeans gained knowledge from many Arab writers. One to note was John Mesue (c. AD 850), who wrote *'De Re Medica.'* Another was Avicenna (c. AD 980–1037), who wrote *'Canon Medicinae.'* Lastly, Ibn Baitar (c. AD 1197–1248) described over 1000 plants in his writings' *'Liber Magnae Collectiois Simplicum Alimentorum Et Medicamentorum' (Petrovska, 2012)*. Known for their extensive knowledge of medicinal herbs and plants, the Arabs influenced European physicians throughout the Middle Ages.

The Age Of Exploration

Since antiquity, Europe and the Mediterranean's appetite for exotic goods from the East has been immense. Many of these goods came from a place called *'The Indies.'* This area included most of South and Southeast Asia, India, and the East Indies, now Indonesia. Between the 13th and 15th centuries, many explorers traveled the world searching for herbs, plants, and the most prized possession—spices.

Some of the most sought-after spices included pepper, cinnamon, and clove from India; cassia, also called Chinese cinnamon, from China; ginger from Southeast Asia; nutmeg and mace, which come from two different parts of the same plant, from Indonesia. Interestingly, before the mid-19th century, Indonesia was the only place where the nutmeg tree thrived.

These are just a few of the many spices that were worth their weight in gold. These exotic goods reached the Mediterranean through a network of far-reaching trade roots. The most famous of such networks is *'The Silk Road.'* Goods could also be accessed via the sea by a route called *'The Maritime Silk Road.'*

Constantinople became Turkey's most powerful holder of goods due to its position as the furthest Western city on *'The Silk Road.'* Egypt held most of the power over trade on *'The Maritime Silk Road'* with cities in Alexandria to the north along the Mediterranean and Berenice in the East at the Red Sea. From there, transported goods went overland throughout Europe. This perplexing situation made the rest of Europe reliant on these cities for exotic goods, including valuable medicinal herbs and plants. Spain and Portugal became particularly vexed by Constantinople and Egypt's stronghold and realized they needed Western access to the Indies. In the early 15th century, it became a race to see who would make it there via the West coast of Africa.

During this time, known as the late Middle Ages (c. AD 1300–1500), exploration was in full swing throughout the known world. Marco Polo's journeys with his family to tropical Asia, China, and Persia between AD 1254 and 1324 increased the international spice trade *(Petrovska, 2012).* Polo noted sesame oil in Afghanistan, ginger and cassia plants in Peking, and abundant pepper, nutmeg, clove, and other growing plants in Java and the China Sea. Furthermore, Polo even witnessed 10,000 pounds of pepper being loaded into Hangchow, a heavily populated city, and reported loads of cinnamon, pepper, and ginger on the Malabar Coast of India.

The exploration of *'The New World,'* America, brought another influx of medicinal herbs and plants to Europe. Although there is an argument over who discovered the Americas first, history can not deny Christopher Columbus' role. On November 6, 1492, one account states that Columbas' men witnessed the drinking and smoking of two herbs that would later significantly impact the world of pharmacology *(Worth Estes, 1995).* On his second voyage, on the *'western route to the East'* (e.g., the indies), a royal physician Diego Chanca accompanied Columbus in 1493. Chanca would introduce capsaicin (red pepper) and allspice into Spanish cooking.

During the fourth expedition in 1503, Spaniards noted seeing the Panamanian natives chewing on one particular herb. This account is likely the first introduction of coca to the European world. Historians believe Columbus brought both coca seeds and cacao beans back to Spain. Interestingly, the "coca" and "cacao" plants are sometimes thought to be the same, but this could not be further from the truth. Cacao beans produce chocolate, while later in history, the coca plant would be used to make cocaine. However, the indigenous people would chew on the coca leaves to elevate their mood, aid digestion, and suppress their appetite.

The infamous Spanish Conquistador Hernán Cortés traveled to *'The New World'* in 1519. He witnessed the massive market of over 60,000 people buzzing about purchasing all kinds of goods, including herbs and plants, while entering the Aztec capital of Tenochtitlan. He noticed medicinal and sweet goods, roots, and plants from the land sold in large quantities and noted that there were houses much like apothecaries where people could find herbal concoctions for their ailments *(Worth Estes, 1995)*. His expeditions would later bring about the fall of the Aztec Empire.

While the Spaniards moved throughout the *'The New World,'* Portugal was determined to find a western route to the East. On July 8, 1497, the Portuguese explorer Vasco da Gama set sail down the coast of Africa and rounded the nearly impossible Cape of Good Hope on his journey toward the coast of India. The voyage would take almost two years to complete, and the fruits of his labors paid off as Portugal became the supreme power over the spice trade in Western Europe.

Herbalist Linnaeus' Documents

You may have come across scientific terms of organisms before. Notice how there is a distinct way of naming them. Have you ever wondered why it is done this way? Let me tell you!

A Swedish botanist named Carolus Linnaeus (c. AD 1707–1778) brought about a revelation in the classifications of living things. He became known as *'The Father of Taxonomy'* and produced many books throughout his lifetime. His early publication of *'Species Plantarium,'* May 1, 1753, described and classified the species known at that time, although he did not consider descriptions made elsewhere in other naturalists' work *(Petrovska, 2012)*. His work would take him to levels far surpassing his rivals, and some even call him *'the man who named everything!"*

Linnaeus formulated a binomial system in which the first name would be capitalized and given the genus name. A genus is the root of the scientific terms you might have seen before. At the same time, the rest of the classification would identify other features of the plant, animal, fungi, or bacteria. Linnaeus' system became a practice throughout history but was not officially recognized and agreed upon until 1930.

Discovery & Isolation Of Compounds From Herbs & Plants

Analytical discovery of drugs found in plants started around the 19th century. At the tender age of 22, German apothecary assistant Friedrich Sertürner succeeded in isolating and extracting morphine crystals from tarry poppy seed juice in 1804. Sertürner's studies of the drug would take over the next 13 years of his life. While testing the compound on rats and stray dogs, he would later induce destructive trials on himself and three young boys *(Atanasov, 2015)*. Due to its sleep-inducing qualities, he appropriately names it morphium (morphine) after the Greek god of dreams, Morpheus.

In 1817 he published his complicated works on the isolations of pure morphine, where he noted that a 15-milligram dose was optimal. His prescription eliminated the dangers of overdoses from raw poppy juice. Sertürner's publications would eventually activate curiosity in others to examine natural herbs and plants throughout the rest of the 19th century.

Alkaloids could be isolated from natural sources and would be one of the top areas of research and development. Some to consider are nicotine, caffeine, codeine, quinine, and cocaine. The evolution of pharmaceutical companies traces back to the 19th-century apothecaries that specialized in purifying these compounds. The enterprise of chemical synthesis, wherein natural products are physically and chemically manipulated, took off like wildfire.

The goal of these initiatives in research was to produce high-quality results at a low cost. In 1853, this undertaking proved fruitful, with Salicylic acid becoming the first natural compound completed through chemical synthesis. The extraction and isolation of the mix came from the bark of a willow tree *(Salix)*, from which it gets its name.

Nutraceuticals & Innovative Use Of Herbs & Plants

In the early 20th century, due to many authors' scrutiny, medicinal plant manufacturing methods changed dramatically. Arguments arose about techniques for cultivating and drying medicinal plants. *(Petrovska, 2012)*. There was no absolute consistency or standard of practice, which made the healing action of medicinal herbs and plants different depending on who produced them. Due to this inconsistency, proposals for stabilization methods for fresh plants took effect, especially those with medicinal properties.

Throughout the 20th and 21st centuries, the innovative use of herbs and plants has grown. Nutraceuticals are a critical discovery in this field that deserves a highlight. The founder and chairman of the Foundation for Innovation in Medicine, Dr. S. DeFelice, coined "nutraceutical" in 1989. He combined the terms "nutrition" and "pharmaceutical."

Today, nutraceuticals are characterized in marketing to describe any product derived from food sources that provide extra health benefits in addition to the fundamental nutritional value found in food *(Zeisal, 1999)*. Many products, including herbal supplements, fall under this umbrella category because there are minimal international regulations.

So, you should always remain vigilant and know the background of the companies where you buy supplements! Quality control is a must for anything you put in your body. The old saying goes, *"if you want it done right, you should do it yourself."* That is where this book, *Herbal Remedies for Optimal Health and Vitality,* will guide you toward producing products like herbal capsules as supplements at home.

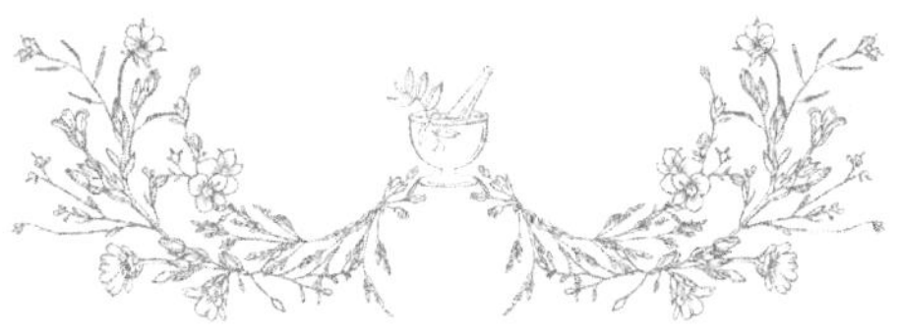

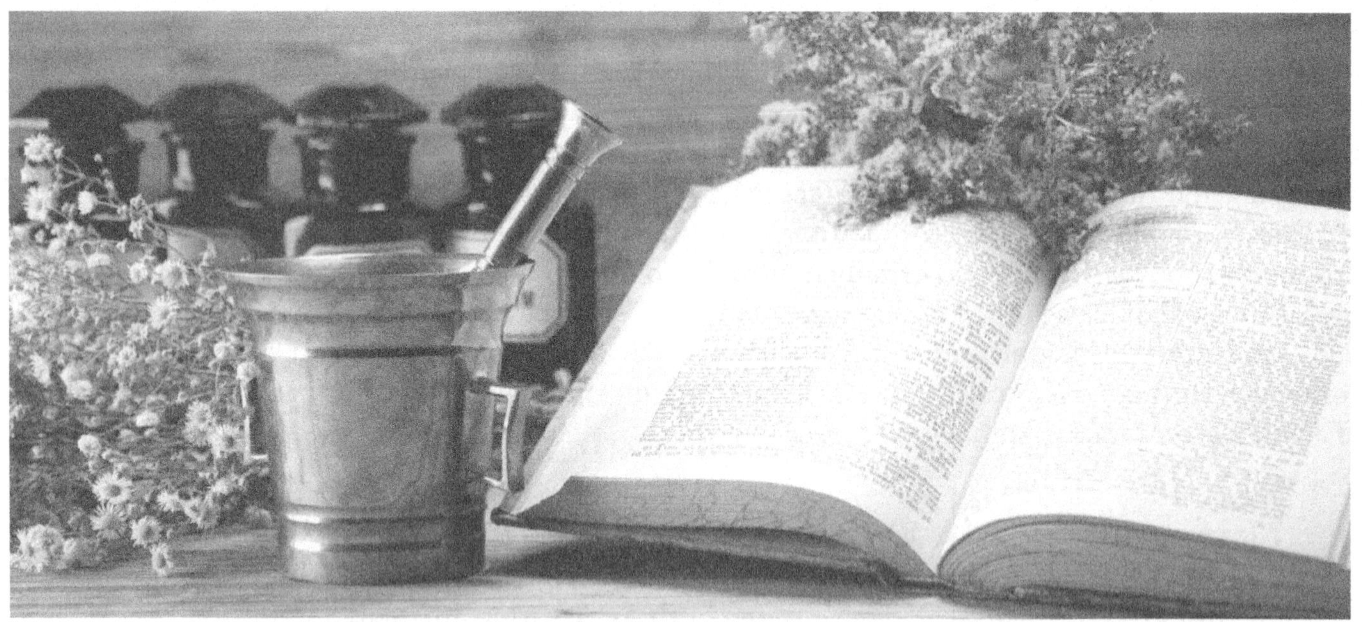

Chapter 2

Herbal Language & Concepts

Are you worried about being confused or intimidated by some new terminologies you will encounter? Going through your journey in herbalism would not be as smooth if you did not have the basic foundations of what you need to know. Do not worry; this chapter will help you!

Here are some herbal language and concepts you might want to look into before starting. Although you may also find this part of the book somewhat dull, if that is the case, feel free to skip ahead. You can always use this chapter as a reference when you run into words or concepts unfamiliar to you.

Herbal Science, Approaches, & Relevant Schools Of Thought

For centuries, different cultures have had countless philosophies about herbal medicine. Some originated from locations based on confounded beliefs, while others were based on specific practices of a group of people.

Allopathy - is synonymous with conventional, modern, or Western Medicine. This system is a medical practice that uses different methods, such as drugs or surgery, to manage symptoms.

Aromatherapy - a topical, inhalation, or oral method of consuming essential oils from medicinal plants to take advantage of its physiologic effect.

Ayurveda - part of the Indian medical system that includes a personalized holistic recommendation for optimal health and vitality. This approach focuses on balancing the three doshas (types of energy) found in everything and everyone: pitta, vata, and kappa.
Eclectic Medicine - used physical therapy practices and medicinal plants during the late 19th century and early 20th century. The practitioners of this have a philosophy founded on "alignment with nature."
Flower Essences - this method infuses flowers with a proportional amount of alcohol, applied topically. Dr. Edward Bach developed this method during the 1930s as he believed flower essences embody a pattern from certain flowers and may rejuvenate an individual's emotional state.
Herbalism - is the art and science of utilizing all sorts of plants and their particular parts and using numerous preparations to support healing and promote overall vitality.
Homeopathy - is a school of thought based on the idea that the body can cure itself, similar to saying that "like cures like." As one thing can cause symptoms in an individual, the same thing given in a minute dose can induce the body to become healthier by training the body's natural defenses.
Indigenous or Tribal Medicine - pertains to practices that transcend generations of applying traditions, ceremonies, rituals, and techniques in botanical approaches. This practice may be unique to a particular group or people in a geographic location.
Naturopathic Medicine - a school of thought that encompasses the scientific, natural, and empirical methods of applying therapeutic strategies that promote an individual's self-healing.
Traditional Chinese Medicine (TCM) - is a plethora of centuries of understanding and practicing various sciences, like using herbs, acupuncture, massage therapy, etc., to correct an imbalance or manifestation of a health problem in an individual. TCM promotes balance between the yin and yang and the body's vital force ('Qi'). It treats the whole person rather than the disease or ailment.
Western Herbalism - traditional Western herbalism constitutes traditions and herbal plant applications from different parts of the world and throughout history. This herbalism also aids modern research in understanding the applications of medicinal plants to allopathy.

Prominent Herbalism Preparations & Delivery

These schools of thought on herbal sciences gave way to innovations in various approaches to extracting and preparing plant-based concoctions and applying them to individuals. Now, you can observe many ways herbal products can be made for home use and at the level of big-time manufacturers.
Acetract/Acetum - a preparation where vinegar extracts valuable compounds from fresh or dried plant materials.
Carrier Oil - oils from plant parts like seeds, kernels, or nuts. These carrier oils are used in diluting other concentrated oils so that you can safely carry the active components of the essential oils onto your skin.
Compress - soaking a cloth or gauze with an infusion or decoction of a liquid herbal preparation applied externally to a particular body part. (See Chapter 8 for more information)
Cream - an emulsion of oil (usually infused with herbs) and water (which may be an infusion or decoction). This preparation makes a product in a semi-solid state. (See Chapter 8 for more information)

Decoction - a method of preparation typically preferred for dense plant parts like roots, barks, berries, seeds, etc., where components are extracted through water and continuous heat supply for around 20–45 minutes. Decoctions are more concentrated preparations as compared to infusions. (See Chapter 8 for more information)
Elixir - a preparation that produces a clear, sweet-tasting liquid with at least one active ingredient. Some commonly added ingredients in elixirs are honey, simple syrup, or alcohol, such as brandy and vodka.
Essential Oil - a process where a distillation process obtains plants' volatile oils and compounds. These oils are commonly used in aromatherapy. (See Chapter 8 for more information)
Extract - a collection of relevant preparation techniques made to concentrate and preserve the active compounds in the plant. Plant extracts include tinctures.
Eyebaths/Eyewash - a gentle preparation made of cold infusions and diluted herb products. Eyebaths are used for bathing parts of the face around the eyes to reduce redness, itchiness, and sometimes, infection. With this preparation, it would be best to ensure that plant material is completely removed or filtered out before use.
Gargle - a liquid preparation, usually anti-inflammatory or disinfectant, where mouthwashes containing active components from plant products are swished in the mouth. (See Chapter 8 for more information)
Gel - a semi-solid preparation where a solid substance undergoes colloidal dispersion with a liquid or gas. You can come up with a jelly-like consistency with this preparation.
Glycerite - a liquid herbal preparation where the plant substance is dissolved or mixed with vegetable glycerin.
Infused Oil - an oil where herb compounds are extracted through infusion over a relatively long time, which varies from hours to weeks. Sometimes, heat is applied in the process. (See Chapter 8 for more information)
Infusion - a preparation method typically preferred with softer plant parts like leaves or flowers, where components are extracted through water. (See Chapter 8 for more information)
Liniment - a topical preparation where plant components are infused with alcohol.
Lotion - a liquid preparation containing water, alcohol, or both. This preparation emulsifies or suspends some insoluble plant products so that they can be topically applied to the skin.
Maceration - a method of extraction where herbs and plant parts are soaked in a menstruum, or solvents, such as vinegar, ethanol, or vegetable glycerin. The mixture sits at room temperature for a long time, depending on the solvent used.
Marc - refers to the solid plant product used in tinctures or extractions.
Percolation - a liquid preparation where you gradually descend liquid, such as water or alcohol, through dried plant material. Plant materials used here are usually powdered and constantly filtered during the process.
Plaster - a particular medicated or protective dressing made by spreading powder and moistened herbs onto a cloth that is then applied to the desired area. It also helps to wrap the plaster in plastic for added protection, which also helps trap body heat, making it more effective.
Poultice - a preparation where you topically apply solid plant materials like powders or leaves mashed with water. When used, the poultice can be contained in the area by placing a suitable material like cloth or bandage. (See Chapter 8 for more information)
Salve - is a preparation that combines oil and wax, infused with herbs. This produces a semi-solid, fatty herbal concoction that is externally applied. (See Chapter 8 for more information)

Steam Inhalation - a type of hydrotherapy where various herbs are infused in a pot or kettle and breathed deeply in, primarily used to alleviate sinus and mucus congestion. (See Chapter 8 for more information)
Suppository - a preparation inserted into the rectum or vagina to deliver a localized herbal mixture. Suppositories melt when introduced to body temperature, which aids the delivery of the herbal mixture's active components.
Syrup - an herbal preparation where concentrated decoctions are mixed with honey or sugar to make a spreadable paste. (See Chapter 8 for more information)
Tinctures - refer to the liquid extracts of plants that are specifically macerated (soaked) in alcohol, but you can also use apple cider vinegar for a non-alcoholic approach. Average tinctures are made with 1 part fresh herb weight to 2 parts liquid volume (1:2), or a ratio of 1 part herbs to 5 parts liquid volume for dried herbs (1:5). With concentrated mixtures, prepare the fluid extracts by following a 1:1 ratio. (See Chapter 8 for more information)
Tisane - this preparation refers to infusions of dried or fresh herbs commonly used as a medicinal drink.

Plant Parts & Other Essential Herbal Terminologies

Most of the time, targeted active components are only found in specific plant parts. Therefore, knowing how to refer to different parts of plants is essential!
Aetheroleum - refers to some of the distinctly obtained essential or volatile oils from plants.
Aerial - refers to the parts of the plant above the ground, including fruit, flowers, seeds, leaves, stems, and petioles.
Balsamum - is a resin and volatile oil solution produced by specialized plant cells.
Bulbus - refers to a plant's bulb or underground bud. Here, you can see shoots or roots grow.
Cortex - refers to the plant's bark obtained from its root, stem, or branches.
Flos - refers to a plant's flowers. The flos may contain a single flower or entire inflorescences, including the head, panicle, spike, etc.
Folium - refers to a plant's leaves.
Fructus - refers to a plant's fruit or berry. The term fruit can further be defined as the ripe ovary of a flower-bearing seed.
Gum Resin - refers to secretions from plants that consists of resin mixed with gum.
Herbs - refers to seed-bearing plants that do not have woody stems. These plants die down to the ground after flowering.
Lignum - refers to the woody stem of a plant or secondary thickening.
Oleum - refers to a fixed oil preparation pressed from plant parts.
Pericarpium - refers to a fruit's peel or rind.
Pyroleum - refers to tar that can be extracted from dry and distilled plant parts.
Radix - refers to the plant's root. The term radix may also bear the same meaning as a rhizome.
Resina - a resin secreted by a plant or obtained by distilling its balsamum.
Rhizome - refers to a creeping horizontal stem. This portion is a root-bearing part of the plant.
Stamen - is a plant's seed that is removed from its fruit. (Male reproductive organ in plants)
Strobiles - a cone-like fruit with tightly layered sporophylls on a central axis.

After becoming familiar with the different plant terminologies, it is now essential to understand the term vitality. Vitality is defined as being able to live and grow. Depending on its use, its overall meaning is dynamic. In our context, a vital individual has a holistic physical and mental state.

While one of the benefits of a herbalist lifestyle is making you feel holistically healthy and vital, not everything is a road to vitality. You may need to change your lifestyle, and achieving a sound mind and positive energy takes time.

Because of Mother Nature's fantastic compounds, medicinal herbs and plants do wonders for your body. If you ever feel overwhelmed by knowing about herbal concepts, this chapter is the quick overview you need. Now, it is time to dig a little bit deeper.

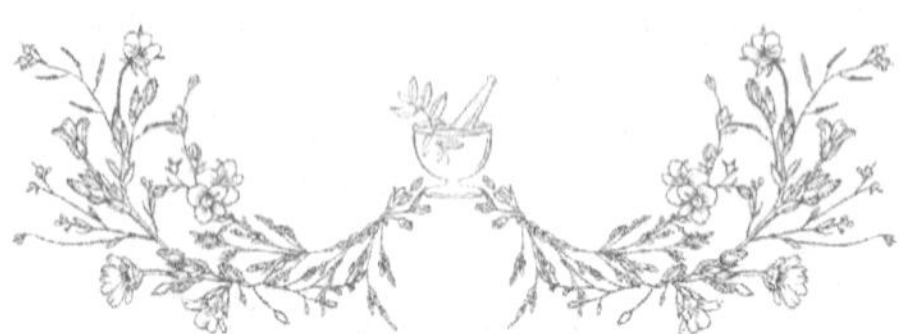

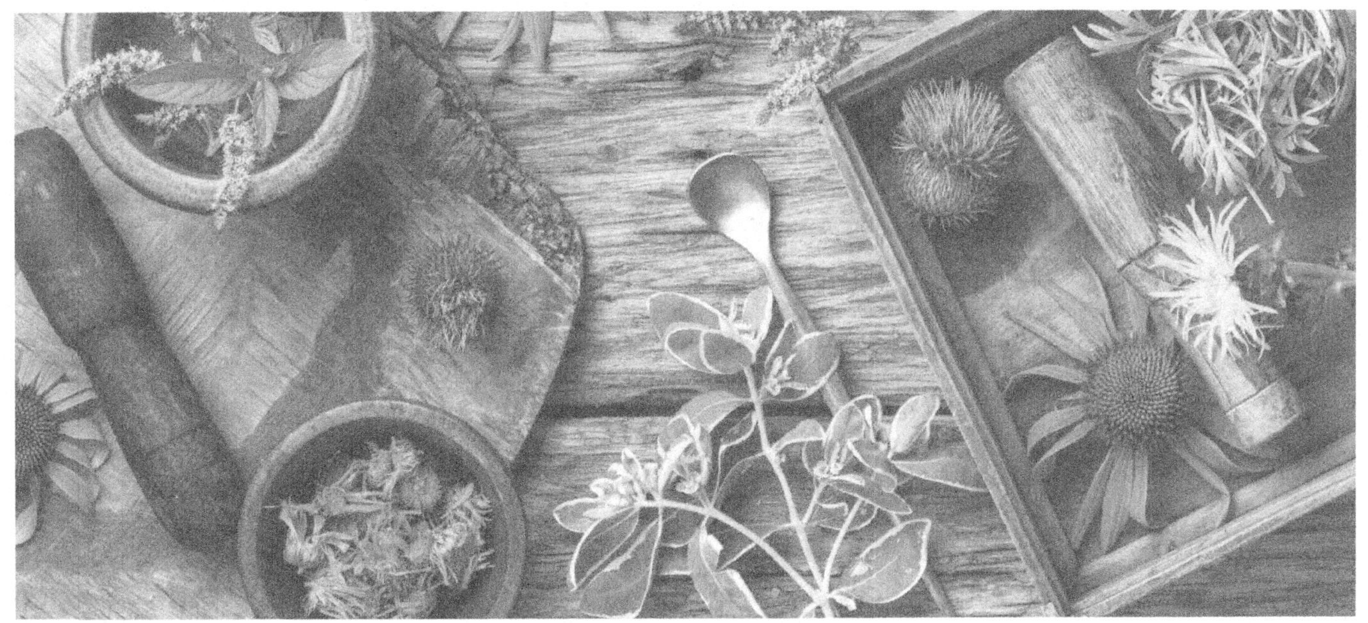

Chapter 3

How Herbs & Plants Work

Humanity's history of introducing, using, and innovating herbalism can show us so many insights. First, humans tend to seek the help of natural ingredients to manage symptoms and eventually find a more sustainable lifestyle that is holistic. Second, herbalism is something that numerous cultures have adapted despite having minimal to almost no contact with each other. These insights prove how valuable herbs and plants are to nearly all locations around the globe.

One of the most common reasons for living an herbal lifestyle would be its affordability and accessibility. Also, it presents little to no side effects if used correctly and could even help ease issues caused by the side effects of synthetic medications.

In reality, individuals have many more reasons to seek a more natural and herbalist lifestyle. Regardless, studies cannot deny that traditional medicine remains essential in healthcare and can serve people who want to take a more holistic approach *(Evans et al., 2007)*. It is almost impossible for herbalism to be "outdated" anytime soon!

Aside from these, did you notice herbalism's practice never stopped decades into the modern era? The traditions of our ancestors are still relevant today. Furthermore, modern medicine has not overlooked the potential of herbs and plants.

Around 25% of modern drugs prescribed to individuals globally have active components derived from plants *(Benzie & Watchtel-Galor, 2011)*. For example, herbs are used for inflammation, impaired immune system, heart problems, and depression. Research in a bulletin by The World Health Organization showed how China effectively used Traditional Chinese Medicine to promote health in acute respiratory syndrome cases. The study also shared how Africa used Hypoxis hemerocallidea (African potato) to manage wasting symptoms of HIV, such as weakness and progressive weight loss *(Tilburt & Kaptchuk, 2008)*. Herbs and plants can still promote health concerns in the modern era.

How are all these accomplishments possible? Plants have particular compounds, sometimes called constituents, that enable them to deliver all these effects. The history of many well-known medicines shows how it is done. Morphine, a pharmacologically active product, was made by extracting opium from the breadseed poppy *(Benzie & Watchtel-Galor, 2011)*. This breakthrough proved that an individual could purify active compounds and use them in precise dosages. Even the discovery of penicillin came from the innovative purification of plant compounds *(Li & Vederas, 2009)*. The contributions of herbs and plants make them an essential part of our modern pharmaceutical modalities.

Aside from simply extracting them, there are many forms the various plant compounds can take. To illustrate, you may have seen herbal supplements in capsules, tablets, or powdered form. Similarly, you can infuse teas or make herbal syrups to add to soda or your favorite cocktails. Likewise, topical applications through oils, ointments, and creams are also possible.

Active compounds from these fantastic plants give us many benefits. Understanding what these compounds can do and how they do it is essential. With this information, the appreciation of the wonders of herbalism will deepen. Now, let us look at some of these active plant ingredients that have proven to be very useful.

Common Active Ingredients In Herbs & Plants

Anthraquinones

Some plants have more distinct dyes compared to others. Anthraquinones are compounds found in plants that give color, making them a widely utilized natural dye or pigment. In addition to their vibrant colors, anthraquinones can also possess some physical effects on the body. Anthraquinones are potent laxatives because they stimulate certain parts of the gastrointestinal tract *(Portalatin & Winstead, 2012)*. Depending on the compound's use, it can be antifungal or antiviral.

Some plants with very high levels of anthraquinones include aloe, rhubarb, and senna. Pharmaceutical companies utilize senna to extract sennosides, the prime ingredient in over-the-counter constipation medications *(Seeff et al., 2013)*. So, anthraquinones are widely available and undoubtedly effective!

Alkaloids

Alkaloids are compounds with different chemical structures but are all composed of nitrogen molecules *(USDA, n.d.)* This molecule is said to help alkaloids deliver health benefits to the body. When alkaloids are obtained from plants, they exert different health benefits, and scientists have exhausted studies to gather as much knowledge as possible about them.

All scientific jargon aside, alkaloids affect the body's physiological actions. They can help prevent neurodegenerative diseases like Alzheimer's, Huntington's, and Parkinson's *(Hussain et al., 2018)*. The potential of alkaloids is continuously being discovered in modern medicine.

Bitters

The grouping of active ingredients in herbs and plants is not always scientific or technical. Take, for example, the bitters. This group is made of numerous plant species called bitter because of their inherent bitter taste.

Eating something bitter is not always the best experience. However, the bitter taste of these plants stimulates the salivary glands and digestive organs *(USDA, n.d.).* Consequently, this can help improve appetite because of the increased salivation and can also help strengthen the digestive system.

Cardiac Glycosides

As the name suggests, this group of active compounds can promote heart wellness, vitality, and blood circulation. Its diuretic effects may urge urination, but this helps promote healthy and fluid-free tissues in the body.

Coumarin

This naturally active compound is present in plants like sweet clovers, pubescent angelica, and ashitaba. Coumarin is fantastic because of its outstanding drug potential. It can produce stable compounds with very low toxicity. There is evidence supporting coumarin's ability to defend against viruses like HIV or influenza, and it even has some impact on multifactorial diseases like Alzheimer's and Parkinson's disease *(Mishra et al., 2020; Stefanachi et al., 2018).* This action is possible because coumarin safely works on the body's cells and targets harmful pathways.

Cyanogenic Glycosides

Cyanogenic glycosides are cyanide-based glycosides. You may be familiar with the destructive nature of cyanide but do not worry; it is the dosage that makes the poison! A toxic amount is between 0.5 and 3.5 milligrams based on body weight. This active compound can promote muscle relaxation and soothe dry coughs when taken in small quantities.

Like other active compounds, cyanogenic glycosides can be found and extracted from plants. It is generally found in the edible parts of apples, apricots, plums, and peaches. The seeds of these fruits contain the highest amount of this compound, but it is also found in the bark of wild cherry trees, barley, and the leaves of elderberries.

Flavonoids

Flavonoids are one of the most widely found active components in plants that exhibit a wide range of health-promoting benefits. Flavonoids can be found in onions, grapes, tea, berries, and vegetables like broccoli. So, what can this compound do?

Flavonoids are excellent because they can help regulate the body's cells and defend them from free radicals. These free radicals are unstable molecules that harm healthy cells. Flavonoids are also natural antioxidants, have anti-inflammatory action, and may help decrease the risk of heart problems or diabetes *(Watson, 2019).* Adding flavonoid-containing plants or food to your diet can help sustain a holistic lifestyle.

Glucosinolates

If we think about green, leafy vegetables, it is impossible not to have some form of active compounds in them. Glucosinolates are compounds that contain sulfur and are found in broccoli, brussels sprouts, kale, cauliflower, cabbage, radish, and much more. Remember that vegetables containing glucosinolates have a bitter taste and a slightly pungent smell.

Glucosinolates can help promote a holistic lifestyle because they may help reduce cancer risks and protect the body from heart attacks and stroke *(Lehman, 2021).* Even though many vegetables contain glucosinolates, cooking them too long can destroy myrosinase. Which is an enzyme that helps convert glucosinates into the body's metabolism.

Minerals

Herbs and plants are nourished by the soil, sunlight, and water based on their individual needs. Each plant absorbs different levels of mineral contents from the dirt, and as a result, we acquire the benefits of their mineral contents. Minerals are necessary substances in making the human body healthy. Some familiar minerals are calcium, potassium, sodium, magnesium, iron, zinc, and iodine.

In medicine, mineral content is the main factor that provides a medicine's effect *(USDA, n.d.).* For example, minerals are great at repairing the body's connective tissues, and horsetail is a plant with high mineral content. Therefore, horsetail may aid in repairing connective tissues related to arthritis issues.

Phenols

Phenols are an abundant component in plants. This active compound allows the shrub to protect itself from plant-eating insects. Some phenol-containing plants you may be familiar with are wintergreen, willow, and the entire mint family.

Aside from that, phenols are well-known as potent antioxidants *(Dull & Mumper, 2010).* Powerful antioxidants like phenols can help lower one's susceptibility to many conditions by neutralizing the effects of oxidative stress. Oxidative stress causes excess free radicals to be produced in the body, which may lead to chronic inflammation or viral infections. Phenols have been studied for their antiviral, anti-inflammatory, and antiseptic benefits.

Polysaccharides

Polysaccharides are unique active compounds found in all herbs and plants. When looking at the chemical structure of this compound, it has numerous units of connected sugar molecules. This configuration gives the gummy texture to plant parts like barks, roots, or leaves. This sticky substance is a polysaccharide and exerts several health benefits when used correctly *(USDA, n.d.).* The components of polysaccharides make it possible to help dry skin and mucous membranes.

Proanthocyanidins

Plants and fruits come in different colors, partly due to the active components that we find in them. Proanthocyanidins are active compounds that give red, blue, or purple hues to fruits and flowers. Aside from the pigments from proanthocyanidins, they offer sustainable health protections supported by science *(USDA, n.d.).* Red grapes and berries, like hawthorn and blackberries, offer proanthocyanidins that may promote healthier blood circulation in the body.

Saponins

Saponins are a familiar word encountered when talking about soap. This is because saponins are active compounds in plants that can lather when submerged in water, making them a great soap ingredient. You can extract this from saponin-rich plants like agave, wild yam, and lilies.

This soapy ingredient has many uses, and we have numerous ways of producing valuable products with them. Saponins may also boost the immune system, promote better metabolism, and help conditions like diabetes or obesity *(Desai et al., 2009).* As long as saponins are extracted correctly and taken in the correct doses, they are safe!

Tannins

Like phenols, tannins are active components that prevent insects and other animals from eating the plant. All plant leaves, tree bark, roots, and some fruits have tannins. They are natural antioxidants, anti-inflammatory agents, and antibacterial compounds that may protect the body from heart problems, diabetes, and neurodegenerative problems *(Boyers, 2021).* This compound provides truly well-rounded and holistic health benefits.

Some herbs containing the highest tannins are green and black tea, yerba mate, oregano, and coca. Even though green and black teas have the most elevated amounts of tannins, all tea has some of this incredible compound.

Vitamins

Of course, this active compound list will not be complete without vitamins. Plants and herbs have many vitamins in them. Unlike plants, which can synthesize their vitamins, animals and humans insufficiently form vitamins in their bodies. Therefore, they must ingest foods high in this active compound to get the sufficient amount needed to survive.

Most fruits and vegetables are rich in vitamin C and beta-carotene. Some less prominent plants like rose hips, watercress, and buckhorn contain higher vitamin B, C, and E levels *(USDA, n.d.)*. Different vitamins focus on giving a particular health benefit.

Volatile Oils

Volatile oils are derived from plant tissues. They are characterized by their failure to saponify and their volatility, meaning the tendency to vaporize. These oils can be distilled because of their ability to evaporate when they are exposed to the air. Steam distillation is the main form of natural volatile oil extraction.

Extracting volatile oils is one of the most significant aspects of herbalism. They produce essential oils that are used for many different purposes. However, volatile oils do not have one specific compound and cannot be attributed to one mechanism that benefits the body. They are a complex grouping with uses that vary from topical application to inhalation methods.

Herbal Actions

Herbalism is fascinating because it provides our bodies with specific actions with minimal harmful effects. As the previous section shows, herbs and plants contain particular active ingredients. These ingredients induce herbal actions. Despite the complex body processes, herbalism always finds a way to give us a specific herbal action we may need.

It is also prudent to understand that herbal actions do not have a fixed intensity of effects. For instance, plants like foxglove and belladonna exert powerful herbal actions, but in contrast, mint or chamomile have gentle actions *(Weiss, 2001)*. This difference does not mean one is less effective than the other; it is just that "gentle" herbal actions do not instantly produce drastic body effects. The following is not an exhaustive list, but are some of the most common herbal actions:

Adaptogen

The root word for adaptogens is "adapt." Herbs with this property help us improve our ability for stress adaptation as they promote better vitality. From a technical perspective, adaptogens affect the endocrine system by modulating balance in the body and boosting the immune system *(ABC, n.d.)*. The adaptogenic properties of herbs and plants help support our body's adaptation to the environment.

Alterative

Better organ function is promoted by the removal of our body's wastes. Some of these wastes include damaged cells, chemicals we absorb from the environment, or additives in our food. Alteratives promote healthy body systems, especially the digestive tract, circulatory, and lymphatic systems. These systems are the body's primary ways of removing waste.

If waste is not removed efficiently, expect symptoms like fatigue or possible infection *(Hillsborough, 2020)*. That is where alteratives prove to be beneficial. This herbal action can help promote vitality in the body by better removal of waste through increasing digestion, purifying the blood, and helping drain the lymphatic system.

Analgesic

Hearing the word analgesic, do you immediately think of painkillers? You would be correct! Analgesic herbs may be localized, meaning a particular herb works only on one body area (only on the skin or joints) *(Hillsborough, 2020)*. Still, this pain-relieving action's advantage may help avoid the potential side effects of potent pain-killing pharmaceutical medicines.

Anticatarrhal

Anticatarrhal reduces the inflammation of mucous membranes of the throat, which may help with respiratory conditions *(ABC, n.d.)*. Plants with this herbal action thin out and reduce mucus build-up in the upper and lower respiratory systems. They can also support the healing of infections in the tonsils, inner ear, and sinuses; furthermore, anticatarrhal helps promote healthy adenoids, part of the lymphatic system.

Antihelminthic

There are instances when the body cannot fight off parasites. Instead, the parasite dwells within the body and sucks off essential nutrients from its host. Some herbs can fight the parasites off because of their anthelmintic properties. Anthelmintics kill or expel parasites like worms from the gastrointestinal tract. Currently, the terms vermifuge, anti-parasitic, and anthelmintics are interchangeable.

Anti-inflammatory

The body develops an inflammatory response to fight an ongoing infection by trying to naturally heal, recover, and reach equilibrium *(Raman, 2021)*. However, if this response gets more destructive to the body rather than protective, it threatens health and wellness. Plants with anti-inflammatory properties can reduce the inflammatory markers in the blood, subsequently diminishing the inflammation.

Antimicrobial

Every day, numerous harmful microbes enter the body and can cause illnesses. These harmful bacteria or fungi are picked up from the environment or other people. Antimicrobial herbs work on microbes by preventing their growth and reproduction in your body *(Hillsborough, 2020)*. Our bodies are constantly in contact with billions of these tiny microbes. They are all around us, and we can not get away from them, but antimicrobial herbs can provide essential functions to help us fight off potential infections.

Antioxidant

The term antioxidant is rather well-used in herbalism. Based on the name, antioxidants fight against oxidants, also known as free radicals, in our bodies. So, what are these oxidants, and why do we need to address them? Our bodies encounter toxins through various means, including smoke, pollution, and processed foods. Unfortunately, too many of these will weaken immunity and degrade cells *(Hillsborough, 2020)*. So, antioxidant herbs can fight these free radicals and prevent harmful damage to the body.

Antispasmodic

Antispasmodics, also called spasmolytics, can help with spasms or cramps in the body, but this action is not limited to muscle cramps! Herbs with antispasmodic actions also help with anxiety, irritability, and emotional and musculoskeletal stress *(Martinez-Perez et al., 2018)*. Some well-known herbs with antispasmodic benefits are opium poppy and belladonna extracts.

Astringent

Astringents can be found in some skin care products that promote the reduction of inflammation and acne and, most notably, tighten skin *(Chertoff, 2019).* Have you noticed that your skin feels tight when you use an astringent toner? This feeling is because toners are a natural astringent that dries and constricts the pores to draw out impurities like oil and dirt. Witch hazel is a natural skin toner with astringent qualities, although the drying effect of an astringent is not suitable for all skin types.

Carminative

Carminative herbs and plants soothe the digestive system due to their high volume of volatile oils. These very aromatic herbs may help reduce gas and help you feel less bloated. Most carrot and mint family members are carminatives, like peppermint, dill, and fennel. Other carminative herbs include garlic, cinnamon, clove, and nutmeg.

Demulcent

The oily viscosity of demulcents coats and protects mucus membranes. A well-known herb with demulcent action is slippery elm. This herb's gummy and slimy texture helps to cool dry, inflamed skin and mucosa *(Marglin, 2021).* To utilize a demulcent property, apply it topically over the skin. Sometimes, it is used to soothe an inflamed esophagus or gut lining by internal means of application.

Diaphoretic

Diaphoretic herbs help the body sweat more, like how you get sweaty after eating spicy peppers. This sweating mechanism helps the body flush out wastes, increase blood circulation, and even help when you have a fever *(Hillsborough, 2020).* Perspiring can initially make the body feel hot, but this process helps skin cool naturally!

Diuretic

At this point, you may have a growing appreciation for the value of removing waste from the body. Like diaphoretics and alteratives, diuretics promote vitality by helping eliminate excess fluid by urinating *(Hillsborough, 2020).* A build-up of too many bodily fluids may predispose you to kidney problems, diabetes, and high blood pressure.

Emménagogue

Emménagogue are plants that can help stimulate and regulate menstrual flow. This management involves normalizing the body's hormone levels as these herbs affect the liver *(Marglin, 2021).* Liver enzymes can spike in the first phase of the menstrual cycle, and emménagogue can help regulate these enzymes.

Some women have concerns with delayed menstrual cycles. Some possible causes for the delay can be stress, anxiety, hormonal disturbance, and many others. Emménagogue may be precisely the herbal action you need! Note that emmenagogues, especially the strong ones, should be used with caution if you are pregnant since they may cause harm to the fetus.

Expectorant

Expectorants are helpful if you have coughs and have problems expelling mucus. This action helps loosen mucus from mucosal linings in the body to help naturally cough it out and make you feel better. Expectorants can either be stimulating or soothing *(Hillsborough, 2020).* Stimulating expectorants are best used if you produce too much loose mucus and need help expelling it. In contrast, soothing expectorants loosen mucus in irritating and unproductive coughs.

Hepatic

Hepatic is a general term referring to herbs that work on the liver. Hepatic herbs help bile, a substance produced in the liver, to have better flow and tone *(Hillsborough, 2020).* Having an appreciation for the role the liver plays is something to keep in mind! No other organ can induce balance and homeostasis better than the liver; it is vital to keep this organ functioning properly.

Laxative

Laxatives are one of the herbal actions that stimulate bowel movement. This action dramatically helps induce colon movement if you have constipation, nausea, or bloating. This movement is called peristalsis *(McDermott, 2018).* Surprisingly, numerous laxatives sold in the market contain herbal extracts as the active ingredient! Some herbs with this action are buckthorn, rhubarb, slippery elm, and psyllium.

Nervine

As the word somewhat implies, nervines benefit the nervous system. They have actions that vary; some can help stimulate, relax, or strengthen nerves *(Marglin, 2021).* They help soothe the nervous system, bringing balance to the body. Herbs, with this action, may be beneficial for anxiety, insomnia, and stress.

Sedative

Sedatives are actions that promote a calmer mood, soothe the nervous system, and may assist with better sleep. The term sedative is widely used because, from the pharmaceutical perspective, these are used for numerous health concerns. Doctors commonly prescribe them for stress, anxiety, and sleep disorders like insomnia.

Naturally, sedatives are present in plants as well. All sedatives, whether plant-based or synthetic, should be used under the supervision of a doctor. They can be addictive and could lead to other health concerns. Although herbal sedatives tend to have fewer to no side effects, this does not mean you should take them without some consideration.

Stimulants

Do you feel down or sleepy frequently? Then, you might want to get the energy-boosting benefits of stimulants. Stimulants help the body regain energy by improving metabolism, increasing circulation, and delivering an abundance of oxygen to cells *(Hillsborough, 2020).* The unique thing about stimulating plants is that they have significantly fewer side effects than pharmaceutical alternatives.

Tonics

Tonics are herbal actions that offer a generic benefit to the body. Generally, these actions can help cells revitalize with the adaptive energy for holistic health *(Hillsborough, 2020).* Furthermore, other benefits of tonics are their anti-aging effects and potential to balance physical and emotional energies. Tonics are usually used to target one organ or system of the body at a time, unlike adaptogens which work on a more whole-body spectrum.

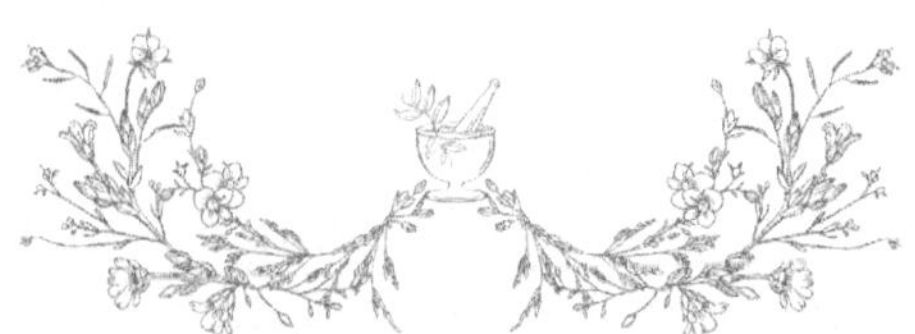

By now, you already have a solid foundation regarding herbalism. As you explore the herbal actions, you might feel more confident about your herbalism journey. As you continue, we will explore a more holistic perspective. In the next chapter, we shall look at several essential pillars for promoting optimal health and vitality with the assistance of herbs and plants.

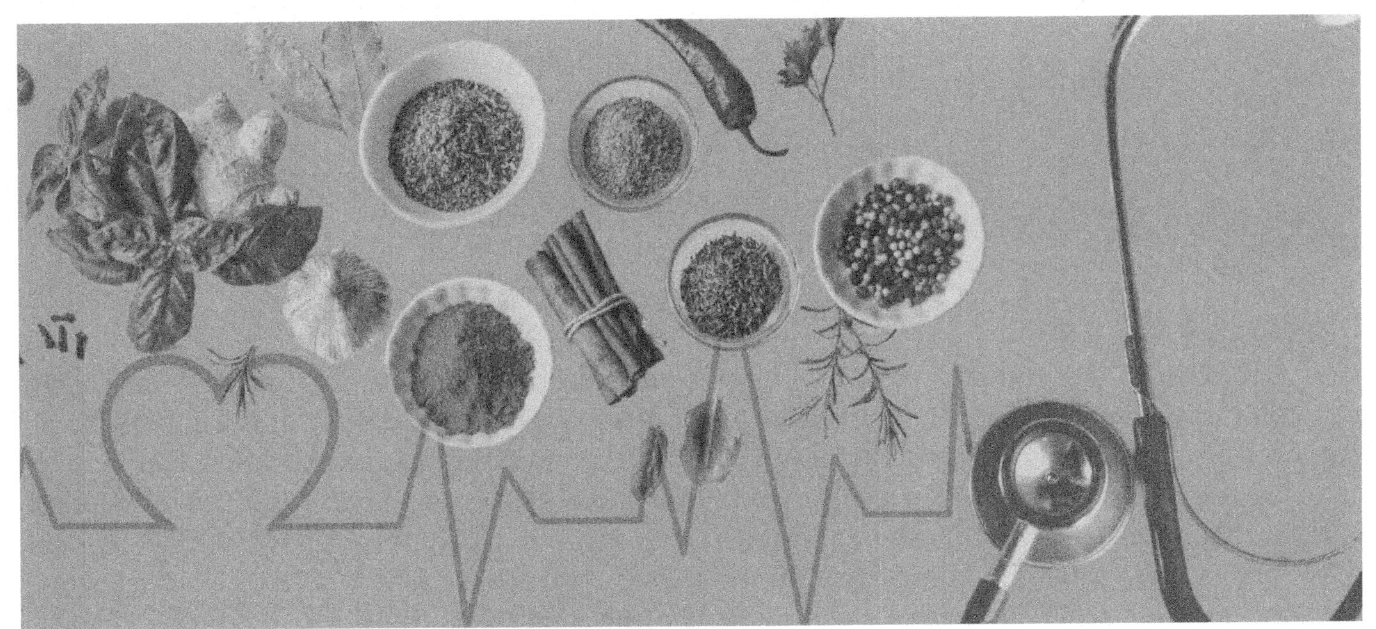

Chapter 4

Herbs, Plants & the 5 Pillars of Optimal Health & Vitality

You may wonder what the five pillars of optimal health and vitality are and what they have to do with medicinal herbs and plants. Herbs work wonders on the body and mind, but they can also affect every aspect of your life if you let them. This chapter will present the fundamental ways medicinal herbs and plants address the significant components of optimal health. You will come to appreciate the wonders hidden inside these gifts from Mother Nature.

Many fresh herbs contain vitamins A, C, K, and polyphenols. Polyphenols are only found in plant-based foods and are plant compounds that have both antioxidant and anti-inflammatory capabilities *(Rautio, 2018)*. Herbs and plants genuinely reach all areas of the body. They support the body's natural ability to heal itself, aid in addressing common ailments, and allow you to achieve overall wellness.

Let us discuss the five health pillars: nutrition, sleep, movement, stress, and connection. Understanding these will help you appreciate herbalism on a deeper level. You will notice how each pillar interconnects with others as they are not stand-alone concepts. For instance, if you do not have good nutrition, you may lose sleep, and if you lose sleep, you may be easily stressed, and so on. Without further ado, here are the five pillars that can aid you in gaining optimal health and vitality.

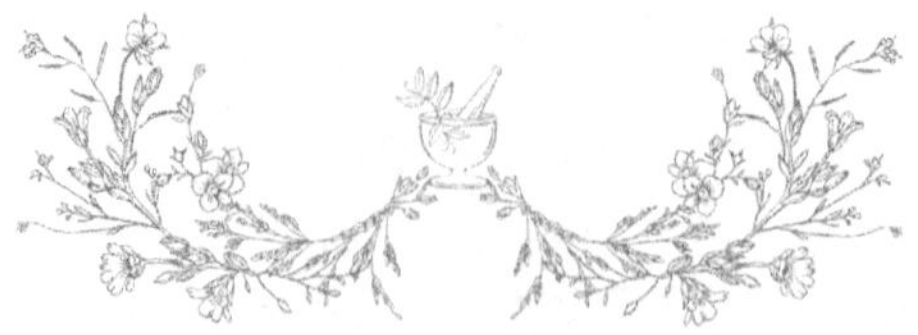

Nutrition

A nutritious diet full of proteins, vitamins, and minerals helps maintain metabolism and keep common ailments at bay. Other things to consider are calorie intake, limited starchy food consumption, and adding plenty of fruits and vegetables to your diet. Fruits and vegetables help to maintain the mineral and vitamin levels required for the body to run smoothly. Garnishing foods with fresh herbs can also aid digestion and absorption of essential vitamins and minerals.

In contrast, some foods may have unwanted consequences if not eaten in moderation. Consuming excess sugar and saturated fat can lead to a laundry list of health issues, including the interruption of nerve cells in the brain. A crucial brain and spinal cord protein, called brain-derived neurotrophic factor (BDNF), is essential in forming new neural growths and synapses. Ingesting high amounts of sugar and fat can cause the brain to produce less BDNF *(Park, 2010)*. Eventually, the lack of this protein can lead to an imbalance in metabolism and many other imbalances in the body.

A healthy, well-rounded diet eaten at the right time will ensure your body gets all the energy, protein, vitamins, minerals, and fiber needed to function correctly. Avoid eating unhealthy snacks in between meals. Nuts and legumes are good sources of protein and are a healthy alternative. Snacking on them between meals can keep you from indulging in junk food.

The human body needs nutrients to work efficiently, but you cannot always get the vitamins and minerals you need from diet alone. There are many herbs and plants we will discuss later that can help absorb the nutrients found in food, but when that is not sufficient, supplements can be a healthy way to help boost the nutrients the body needs.

These supplements are readily available in most local drug stores or herbarium. Be sure to research the companies where you buy products because they are not all created equal. Also, always check with your doctor or nutritionists before starting supplemental therapies. They may be able to point you in the right direction and refer you to trusted products.

Vitamins are another fantastic herbal active component that aids the body in releasing the needed energy from the food you eat. While they do not add calories, they speed up the chemical reactions utilized in digestion and help the body's growth, mental alertness, and nerve functions. Vitamins are involved in many processes enabling the body to use carbohydrates, fats, and proteins for energy and repair.

A nutritious diet must also contain minerals. The mineral content in your diet helps build certain enzymes the body needs to function well. Adequate levels of minerals help optimal nerve function, oxygen distribution, carbon dioxide removal in our cells, and much more.

As you can see, the body is amazingly complex, with systems that need a proper nutritious diet to reach optimal functionality. Here are some herbs and plants that might help in supporting a healthy diet:

Cinnamon: Known for its fantastic flavor, it is an excellent alternative to high sugary foods. It can benefit those with diabetes or anyone looking to reduce their sugar intake. Add a little to a bowl of oatmeal or sprinkle your coffee to curb the need for sweets.

Cayenne Pepper: Cayenne pepper's active ingredient, capsaicin, may curb appetite and burn fat cells. Many hot peppers, like cayenne, have thermogenic effects. Thermogenics is a process where more calories and fat get burned to speed up metabolism *(GrowBigZen, 2021)*. Add a small amount of cayenne powder to a healthy vegetable mix to give a little kick and prevent those afternoon cravings while burning stubborn fat cells.

Thyme: Aside from having some of the highest mineral content, thyme is a fantastic antioxidant that keeps the body free from harmful free radicals.

Parsley: It has an out-of-this-world level of vitamin K. Vitamin K is essential for blood clotting and helps wounds heal.

Asparagus: Known for its high levels of vitamin B, it also helps healthy gut flora as it contains high indigestible fiber insulin that works as a probiotic. When the gut is happy, the nutrients in food are more easily absorbed.

Other herbs that aid gut health are: oregano, bay leaves, cloves, rosemary, slippery elm, and turmeric. These are only a few of the many plants you can add to your daily diet to boost optimal health and achieve your nutrition goals. Little by little, you can raise antioxidant levels, increase thermodynamics, and balance gut health. A well-balanced diet is the first place to start when addressing overall wellness.

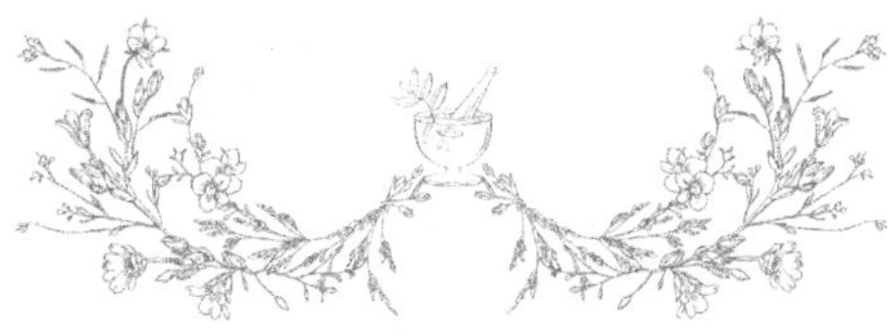

Sleep

John is a medical student and studies for 18 hours a day. Since medical science is a vast subject and retaining information is essential, John is constantly studying. He sleeps only for a couple of hours daily, dramatically affecting his life. Due to lack of sleep, his appetite lowers, and meals often get skipped. Sometimes, the students' cafeteria is unavailable to John when he is hungry, so he ends up munching on unhealthy snacks.

Most students who attend university are like John. They study hard and end up sleeping less. These behaviors negatively affect their bodies' metabolism. Harmful activities to the body are multifactorial, and the combination of these takes a toll on every pillar of optimal health and vitality.

Aside from stressed students, another example is people who work night shifts. They make up their sleep during the daytime, which can cause the same imbalances in metabolism and circadian rhythm (the body's natural sleep-to-wake cycle). Furthermore, their diet suffers, and they either have trouble gaining weight or have difficulty losing it. Overworked people rarely focus on the imbalances that may be causing their health problems.

Tina works two shifts at an e-commerce packaging site. Working two jobs, she rarely has time to stop and eat completely nutritious meals and feels sluggish throughout the day. Tina is sleep-deprived. She has no time or energy to enjoy the money she is making. Aside from this, Tina sacrifices a large part of her body's holistic health.

John and Tina's stories are similar to many people who are not reaching their full potential due to a lack of sleep and nutrition. Chronic sleep loss may increase the risk of heart problems, diabetes, high blood pressure, obesity, and depression. Without sleep, the body cannot function properly, which may affect the amount and types of food eaten. Due to lack of sleep, the hormones regulating appetite get disrupted. This dilemma is especially harmful to young people.

Adolescence is the period in life when kids need to eat healthy food and get plenty of rest to grow up to be healthy humans. Cornell University psychologist James B. Maas, Ph.D., is one of the nation's leading sleep experts. In an interview with the American Psychological Association, he states, *"Almost all teenagers, as they reach puberty, become walking zombies because they are getting far too little sleep" (Carpenter, 2001).* Problems with sleep can start at an early age, but there are ways to help alleviate the restless feeling and return to restful slumber.

Whatever age you are, certain herbs and plants can support healthy sleeping habits and allow you to feel more rested and rejuvenated. The following are a few plants that may aid in good quality sleep:

Turmeric: Turmeric fights inflammation. Adding a spoonful of turmeric powder to a glass of hot milk and drinking it at night before bed can lower inflammation and help you sleep.
Valerian: Valerian is an antispasmodic (pain reliever) that can also increase your coronary blood flow. This root contains more than a hundred components that have sedative effects. The good news is that there are little to no side effects. It is readily available as a tea and can be brewed before bedtime.
Hops: Steeping hops to make a warm cup of tea can be helpful for insomnia. There are also pillows filled with hops that can help with sleep. Sleeping on them can induce sleep as the methyl butanol present in this plant may depress the central nervous system's functions when inhaled *(Foster, 1995).* As the central nervous system calms down, it prepares the body for a good night's sleep.
Chamomile: This plant has numerous applications that date back to ancient herbalism. Studies have shown that chamomile preparations can give mild sedating effects for those who have trouble with sleep, anxiety, and insomnia *(Srivastava et al., 2010).* Sometimes called "the queen of herbs," chamomile can take you into the realms of dreams and give you a good night's sleep.
Passionflower: Passionflower can depress the central nervous system and induce sleep, whether fresh or dried. It reduces anxiety, which in turn helps you fall asleep.

All the herbs and plants mentioned above are sleep inducers with pain and anxiety-relieving properties. When you are free of anxiety and pain, you can have a better night's rest without resorting to pharmaceutical sleeping pills. Brew tea, inhale essential oils from a diffuser, or use essential oils to massage your head and induce sleep.

Massage is a great way to reduce stress and help you sleep better. Apply frankincense or lavender oil and massage your feet before bed. Doing so will relax the mind and has been known to help people fall asleep quickly. Try finding a massage therapist to give you a scalp massage regularly. Choose an essential oil and have them knead it into the scalp to induce blood circulation. The rush of fresh blood to the head helps induce a relaxing state and promotes sound sleep.

Try a full-body essential oil massage to have a more profound effect. While getting a massage, being aware of all the senses can help you relax and become tension-free. A weekly head massage combined with a once-a-month full-body massage can reduce stress and tension, ensuring noticeable improvement in sleeping conditions.

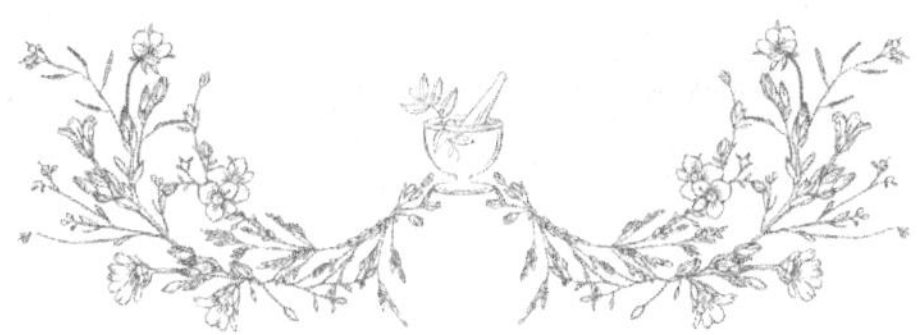

Movement

Optimal health and vitality are inevitable if you pay attention to what your body needs. In addition to nutrition and sleep, the body needs physical and mental movement to maintain overall wellness. Tai Chi, Qi Gong, Pilates, Yoga, weight lifting, and cycling may go a long way in keeping the body agile and relaxed. Whichever form of exercise you choose, adding herbs to your diet can enhance the results and help lower the stress on the body naturally.

Studies have shown that herbal supplements can significantly reduce exercise-induced oxidative stress and enhance muscle performance. When oxidative stress lowers, it speeds up muscle recovery and maintains energy during intense workouts *(Sallami, 2018).* Furthermore, the higher the antioxidant levels in an herbal supplement, the better muscle performance. Herbal tonics and adaptogens support the body during workouts and nourish the body after.

Adding amino acids to your routine can give an extra burst of energy and keep the body going strong throughout a workout. They also help to build and protect protein cells, which is crucial after a hard workout. Consuming the correct plant proteins containing the nine amino acids the body needs to make protein cells is vital.

Some plants that contain these amino acids are buckwheat, soy, and quinoa *(Kubala, 2018).* Amino acids and proteins are the building blocks of life. Herbs and plants can keep you strong as you reach your workout goals. Listed below are a few other herbs and plants that can aid in movement and help get you closer to your workout goals:

Ginseng: Ginseng is one of the most widely studied herbal supplements among leading experts. It has antioxidant qualities to improve physical performance and affects the central nervous system *(Sallami, 2018).* It stimulates cortisol, the hormone that helps our bodies respond to stress.
Arnica: Extracts are available as gels, creams, and homeopathic pills. This herb is highly effective at reducing aches and pains. After a workout, take a few homeopathic arnica capsules or apply the gel to affected achy areas of the body.
Green Tea Extract: Studies have shown that green tea extract (GTE) has helped people prevent weight gain *(Dulloo, 1999).* It also possesses antioxidants, stimulates the central nervous system, and boosts endorphin energy.
Eleuthero: Eleuthero is a rejuvenating root that supports the adrenal glands and boosts endurance before, during, or after a workout. It also helps with mental alertness.
Ginger: Applying ginger directly to the skin after a vigorous workout can soothe muscles. Steep a few ginger tea bags or fresh ginger tea. Allow the tea to cool before applying a compress with a heavy washcloth. Ginger is also high in antioxidants and aids in digestion.
Hemp Oil: Also known as CBD (cannabidiol), hemp oil can relax, de-stress and relieve pain in the

body. The THC present in hemp (0.3%) contains anti-inflammatory properties. Hemp seeds, leaves, stems, and flowers are all useful and have therapeutic properties.

Movement and exercise are essential aspects of optimal health and vitality. If you are not moving, then your body is stagnant. Have you ever seen a puddle of water that is stagnant? It usually has bugs flying around it and a scum layer over the top. Have you ever seen a river or a moving body of water like the ocean? It is powerful, strong, majestic, and beautiful! Which body of water do you want to be? While the above herbs and plants are just a few of the many that can aid in exercise, they are a shortlist to start producing the results you want and assist in keeping you moving.

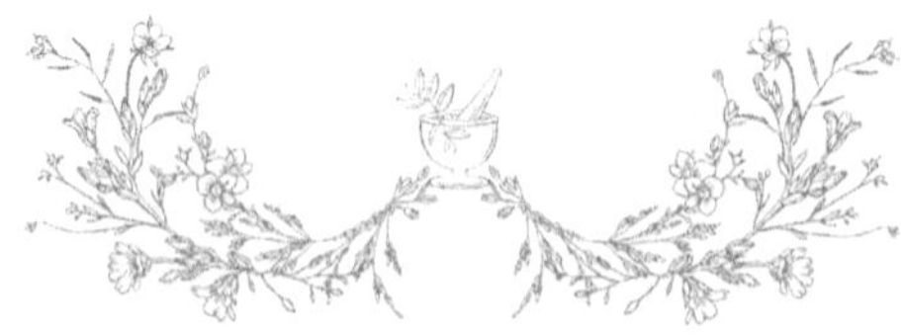

Stress Management

Stress is the body's response to any change that needs an adjustment or answer. It is also the body's way of responding to any demand. The nervous system releases chemicals into the bloodstream when the body feels stressed by an awful experience. This reaction causes the blood pressure to go up due to the sudden influx of energy. When there is no outlet for the extra energy, it remains in the body, causing pain and strain. This tension affects the body and mind, causing an imbalance of hormones.

There are three hormones in charge of the stress response released into the bloodstream from the adrenal glands: cortisol, adrenaline, and norepinephrine. They are responsible for the fight-or-flight reaction when life-threatening situations arise. Adrenaline is also known as epinephrine. Together with norepinephrine, it causes instant reactions like the pounding of the heart and sweaty palms. Cortisol regulates various processes in the body, including metabolism and immune response, and aids the body in responding to stress. Although the response time is slower with cortisol, the body must balance these three hormones for optimal stress management *(Klein, 2013)*. When the body produces too much of one hormone, it must create other hormones to balance them.

A person can be stressed out due to work overload, whereas others may be stressed by having no work. Stress can be irritating, and the problem is that it accumulates and erupts at the most inappropriate time and can cause significant mental breakdowns. There are many reasons for stress. Work, lack of work, career, relationships, financial hardships, and health issues create tension and are perhaps some of the strains you witness daily. Let us look at a situation that walked into my massage studio one afternoon.

Eva lost her job at a bank. Without a steady paycheck and maxed-out credit cards, she immediately freaked out about how the bills would get paid. She checked her savings and realized there was just enough to last her six months. Feeling stressed and panicky, Eva wondered about her survival if she could not get a job fast enough.

Eva was referred to me by a mutual friend. She told me that she had frequent headaches and felt heavy when she woke up in the morning. She was also constipated and, most days, could not eat solid foods. Her diet consisted of mainly drinking coffee and soda throughout the day, and snacking on saltine crackers at lunch was the only solid food she ate. Eva jumped at the slightest sound and cried at the drop of a hat. She was going through extreme stress and anxiety.

I assured her that getting an herbal massage would help free blood flow throughout her body and calm the stress-associated nerves. I also recommended that she drink chamomile tea in the evening to get better sleep so that her body could rest. Adding mint, cilantro, and rosemary to salads would help her flush out the toxins and free her bowel movements.

I gave Eva a relaxing massage with lavender oils. After three sessions, she felt physically and mentally capable of addressing the stressors in her life. Regular massage helped restore her lost health so she could think positively with clarity. Her gut health had improved, and she was eating solid meals again. In three months, Eva got a job and became her usual happy self.

Like Eva, you may look for a simple natural solution to lowering stress levels. Whatever stressors bombard you regularly, herbs and plants can come to the rescue and help you regain optimal wellness. Here are a few that can get you pointed in the right direction:

Lavender: Lavender applied in aromatherapy applications such as massage oils, baths, room sprays, and diffusers can soothe the mind to relieve stress.

Lemon Balm: Lemon balm aids with nerve exhaustion, elevates mood, and reduces anxiety. It has other medicinal properties, such as helping with indigestion, increasing appetite, and promoting sleep.

Catnip: Most people think catnip is only for cats, but it is gentle and effective for everyone, including children and the elderly. It can reduce restlessness and nervousness associated with stress.

Scullcap: Skull cap nourishes the nervous system. It reduces muscle tension and calms the mind.

Holy Basil: Known as one of the essential herbs in India, holy basil promotes vitality and overall wellness. When you feel restored and healthy, you are less prone to stress.

Other herbs that can be helpful when managing stress are: chamomile, hops, passionflower, hemp oil, and valerian. Stress has always been a common aspect of our lives, but it does not mean you cannot do anything about it. Remember, too much stress will lead to unfortunate consequences for your overall health.

Eva was a prime example of how you can alleviate life stressors with the help of an herbal lifestyle. However, your stressors may differ entirely from Eva's, so be aware of what they are. As you can see, many herbs used to manage stress also promote good sleeping habits. All of these pillars are connected, and as such, some herbs will affect multiple areas of optimal health and vitality.

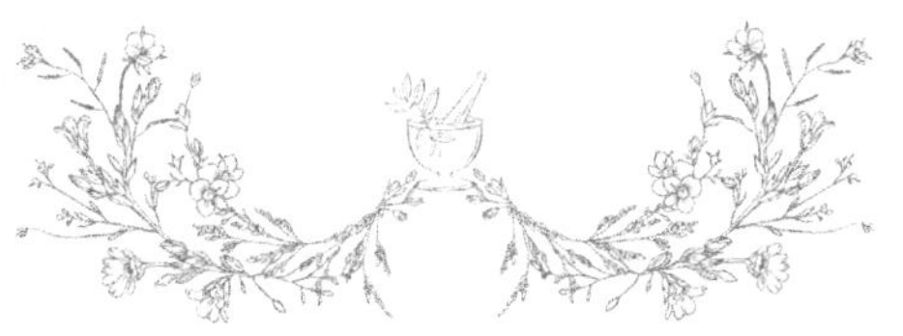

Connection

Connecting with nature and the environment around you can lead to a balance of body and mind. To attain this balance, you must first connect with yourself. It would be best if you found a connection with yourself that is deeply personal. Trust your intuition and know that the beautiful world of herbs and plants is here to guide you on this journey of self-discovery.

Deepen Your Connection With Medicinal Herbs & Plants

First, it is best to have direct contact and experience with plants while observing them in their natural habitat, whether at home or in the wild. There are many medicinal herbs and plants in the wild, but wildcrafting should only be practiced if you are 100% confident in identifying what you are harvesting. Watching them grow from seed to sprouting and full maturity helps create a bond between you and the plant. Take your time with this process, and be patient. Direct contact and experience are some of the most abundant gifts Mother Nature can give you.

The next step to your herbalism journey is to deepen your connection to it. There are numerous ways to do this but do not worry if you find it overwhelming at first. You can try finding the approaches that best fit your skills and resources. For instance, you may try herbal concoctions and remedies, change your diet, or grow an herbal garden. From simple compresses or infusions to tinctures and decoctions, you are sure to develop your connection quickly.

The third way you can connect better to the herbs and plants you use is to incorporate them into your daily life. More consistent use of them will show you their benefits and help you reach optimal health and vitality quicker. Taking remedies causes a physiological sensitivity, and you can feel the plant working in your body. Also, sitting in a meditative state when taking herbs and plants can be beneficial. Set your intention before taking the remedy. Focusing on your mind, body, and spirit during herbal meditations can deepen the healing connection.

If you have friends and family interested in optimal health, ask them to try your remedies and recipes. You can check to see the effects and whether the formula works, but do not be afraid if it does not work. So many budding herbalists stop before they even start because they fear failure. Every herbalist I know has given someone a remedy at some point that did not work. It is all a part of the learning process. If it does not work, you have learned more about that particular remedy and deepened your connection to the plant that made it.

Lastly, you will want to study as much as you can. There are many ways to develop your knowledge of medicinal herbs and plants, from Traditional Chinese Medicine and Ayurveda to Galic and Celtic herbalism. Everything you learn does not need to come from personal experience. The body of knowledge is ancient, and with a bit of research, you are sure to connect with herbs and plants on a deeper level.

You need to have an intimate relationship with your herbs. This relationship will help you appreciate what you have. Herbs and plants are available in most neighborhood nurseries. You can either plant them in a patch of land or keep them in an herb stand indoors close to a window. Tending to different herbs can give you a sense of happiness and joy. As they grow, your appreciation for them will flourish, and you will feel deeply satisfied that you have made a difference in your world.

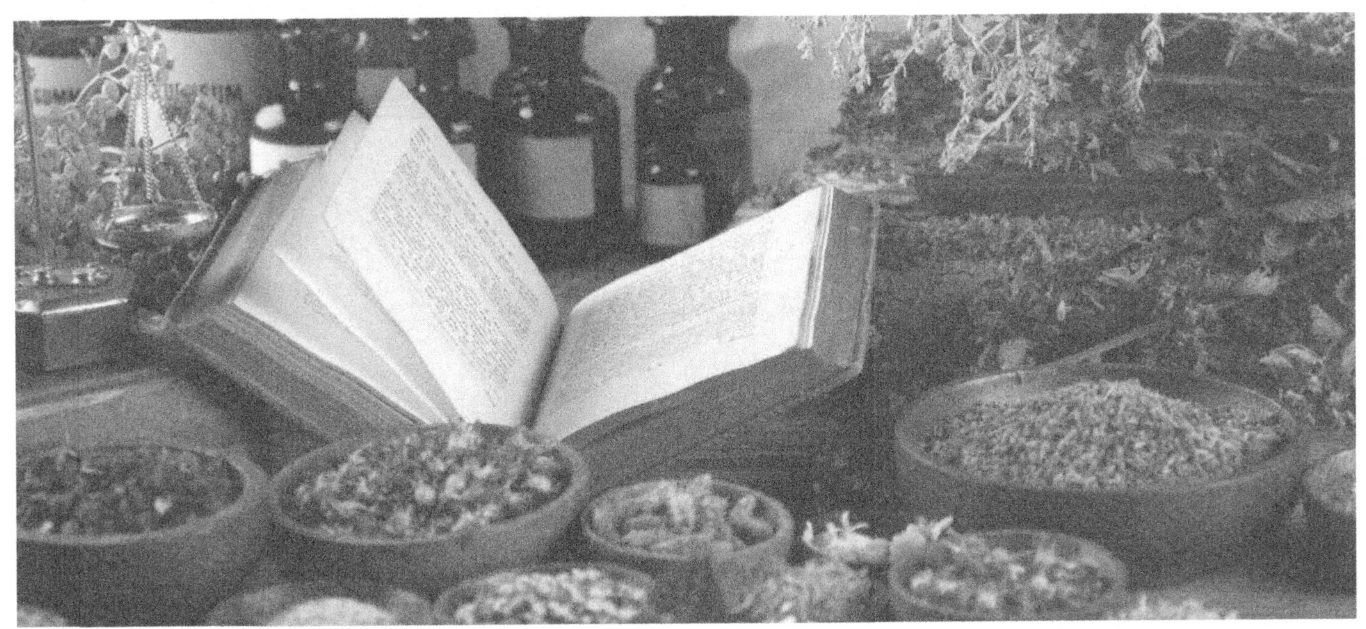

Chapter 5

Top 27 Herbs & Plants for Optimal Health & Vitality

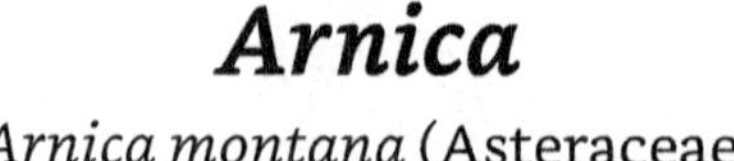

Arnica

Arnica montana (Asteraceae)

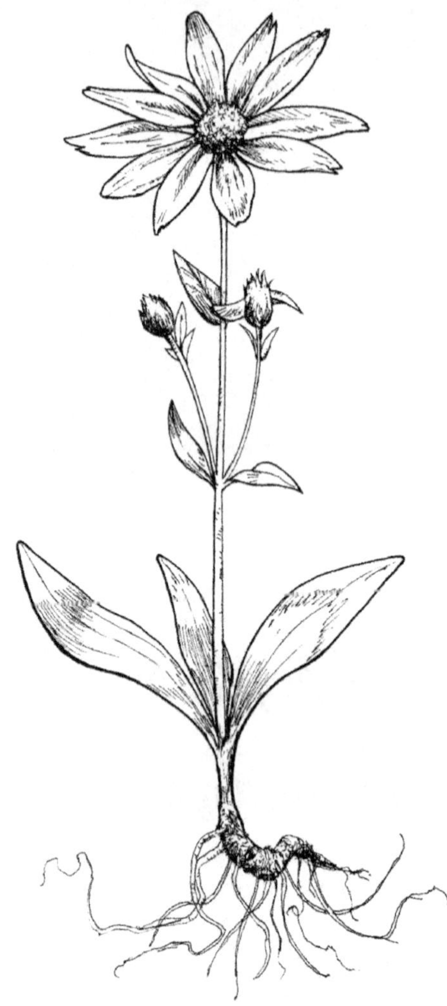

The herbal applications of arnica used by practitioners during early herbalism practices still resemble modern applications today. Its anti-inflammatory and homeopathic capabilities make it suitable for several self-care applications.

When my mom was in an accident and broke her tibia bone, she was bedridden for almost three months. The inflammation in her leg was intense! She began to use arnica gel, and the swelling and discomfort reduced significantly. When she was able to return to work, her knee was still hurting. Arnica ointment was a go-to for her sore muscles and tension. You do not have to break a bone to use this herb! The active compounds in arnica are fantastic for everyday aches and pains.

Description

Arnica is a perennial that grows from a barrel-shaped hairy rhizome and can reach about a foot (30 centimeters) tall. It has a few other names, wolf's bane, mountain arnica, and leopard's bane, but you can identify it by its large yellow flower heads that have a daisy-like appearance. The leaves can be toothed or smooth depending on the species and are often hairy.

History

Arnica has been a known flower with traditional herbal use dating back centuries. As early as

1558, this flower was mentioned in an herbal book by Pietro Andrea Mattioli, a successful author who wrote about botany. He referred to arnica as "Alisma" —the plant's early name. The plant was eventually called arnica by 1625 *(A. Vogel plant encyclopedia, n.d.)* Common uses included aiding individuals who had "fallen" or "hurt themselves while working." During the 18th century, arnica was still one of the leading centers of study since scientists noticed its potential as a homeopathic agent.

Habitat & Cultivation

Arnica is commonly seen growing in sub-alpine areas in North America and several regions of Asia and Europe *(Wong, 2021a)*. Arnica grows in both the sun and shade but prefers alkaline soil. You can see it growing prominently from June through August.

Active Compounds: Carotenoids; Flavonoids; Sesquiterpene lactones such as helenalin; Volatile oil consisting of thymol, mucilage, and polysaccharides

Herbal Actions: Anti-inflammatory; Homeopathic

Parts Used: Flowers and Rhizome

Main Use:

- Accelerates healing
- Muscle and joint pain
- Bruises
- Broken bone inflammation
- Sprains and strains
- Improves local blood circulation
- Helps with reabsorption of internal bleeding

Self-care Use:

- Use arnica ointment on bruises and swelling two to three times a day
- Massage arnica ointment or cream on sprains, strains, or fractures three times a day.

⚠ **Caution!**

- ★ ☠ Arnica is poisonous in concentrated doses. Always dilute! That is why homeopathic remedies are diluted and taken in very small amounts over a short period of time. DO NOT take arnica, in its pure form, internally.
- ★ Arnica should never be applied to broken skin. Dermatitis may occur.
- ★ If you notice any allergic reaction or hypersensitivity to arnica, immediately stop applying it.

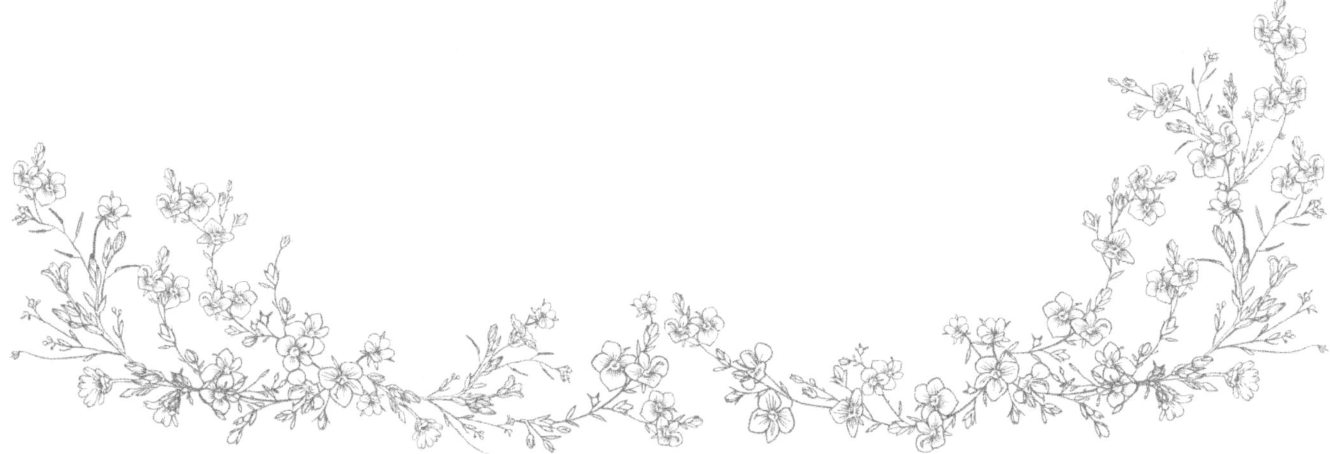

Asparagus

Asparagus officinalis (Liliaceae)

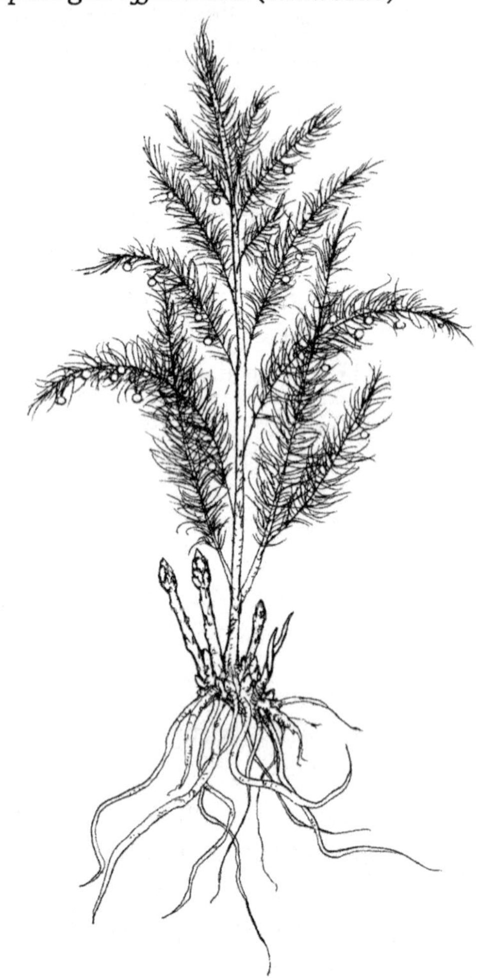

Asparagus is a herbaceous plant cultivated for its shoots or spears, most commonly used as vegetables added to dishes. It also has other benefits due to its low calories and is packed with numerous anti-inflammatory vitamins and minerals.

I was diagnosed with interstitial cystitis, a chronic condition that causes intense bladder inflammation. Heartbroken when the doctor told me not to eat many of the foods I love, I researched what might help. Asparagus was one vegetable that would save the day! I cook this plant to calm my bladder whenever I am in a flare. It almost immediately decreases the inflammation and helps with the spasms that drive me crazy.

Description

The asparagus plant is a perennial that grows to about 6.5 feet (2 meters) tall with leaf fronds that have a needle-like appearance. This plant has rhizomes and underground stems that help it propagate. Bell-shaped flowers grow in singles or pairs with a green-white or yellow color. These flowers produce small bright red berries that are toxic to humans and dogs.

History

Asparagus is a well-cultivated plant from numerous ancient civilizations. The richness of use with this timeless vegetable can be traced back to Egyptian, Greek, and Roman times *(Pegiou et al., 2019)*. The first Egyptian illustration of this plant (4000 BC) is unsure if it holds food or medicinal use since it appears to be an offering. In contrast, the Greeks and Romans had clear evidence of using asparagus as a food source and herbal application. Dioscorides (1st century) noted that asparagus root aided in urine flow and used it to treat kidney issues, sciatica, and jaundice *(Chevallier, 2016)*. Similar herbal applications are noted in Traditional Chinese Medicine as well.

Habitat & Cultivation

Asparagus is native to Northern Europe, North Africa, and Asia *(Pegiou et al., 2019)*, but today it is grown and cultivated in virtually all regions globally. This plant grows best in tropical or subtropical climates, with a preference for medium loamy or heavy clay soils *(Iqbal et al., 2017)*. Asparagus is not the most challenging plant to grow because of its ability to adapt well. Do not harvest the plant for the first two years to give the root system time to establish. One single crown of asparagus can propagate for up to 20 years!

Active Compounds: Asparagine; Bitter glycosides; Flavonoids; Saponins; Steroidal glycosides; Tannins

Herbal Actions: Anti-bacterial; Anti-inflammatory; Antioxidant; Strong Diuretic; Bitter; Mild laxative; Sedative

Parts Used: Rhizomes and shoots

Main Use:

- Urinary problems including cystitis
- Rheumatic conditions
- Hypertension and diabetes: helps flush wastes that accumulate in the joints out of the body in the urine.
- Promotes healthier organs

Self-care Use:

- Bladder infections
- Probiotic aids in good gut health

⚠ **Caution!**

- ★ Asparagus is not advisable for anyone suffering from kidney disease.
- ★ ☠ DO NOT eat the berries! They are poisonous to humans, dogs, and cats. The raw shoots are also mildly toxic, so be sure to cook before consuming.

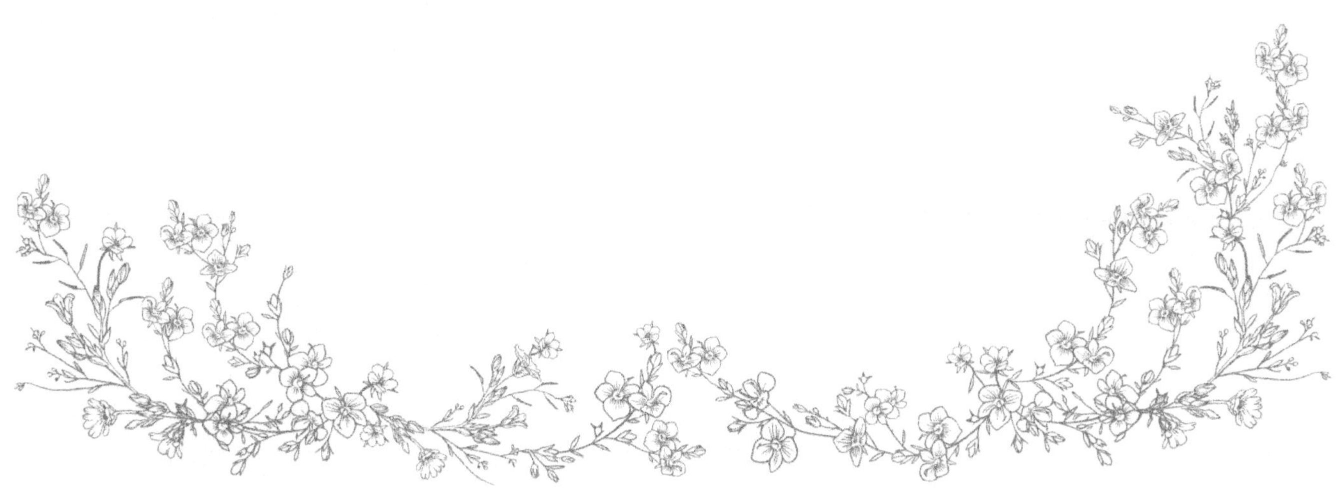

Bay Leaf

Laurus nobilis (Lauraceae)

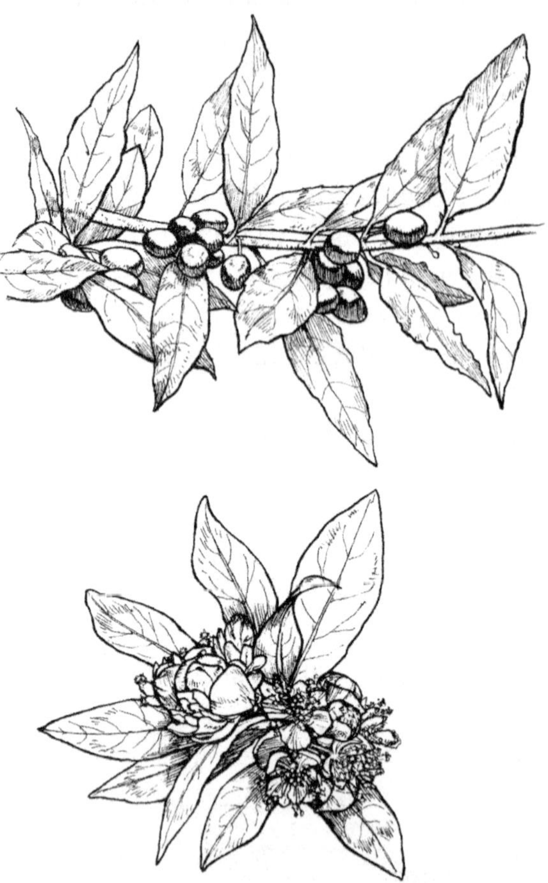

In addition to the delicious flavor that bay leaf can add to your cooking, it also provides health benefits. The traditional use of bay leaf includes alleviating rashes and rheumatism because of its tonic and anti-inflammatory effect and massive antioxidant content.

I have many massage clients that have arthritis. One comes to mind that was suffering from rheumatoid arthritis for years. I suggested she take baths infused with a bay leaf decoction I prepared. When baths were not an option, I gave her a bay leaf-infused oil to apply to the affected areas. She used to come for a massage every two weeks, but after applying these simple bay leave applications, she now comes in every six weeks for a maintenance massage. She now makes her bay leaf decoction and infused oil at home instead of having me make them for her.

Description

Bay leaf is also referred to as Laurel leaf or Bay Laurel. This perennial plant is an evergreen shrub or tree that grows to about 65 feet (20 meters) tall. The leaves are shiny and elliptical-shaped, and the extended branches are olive green. The leaves hold almost all of the plant's value, as they are the most widely used part of the plant.

History

Bay leaves were cultivated even during ancient times, and this common kitchen ingredient carries a rich history. The most common historical use of bay leaves is during the ancient Greeks' time. Old Greek athletes and other notable personalities adorned their heads with bay leaf crowns. *(Britannica, n.d.)*. Apollo and his son Asclepius, the Greek gods of medicine and healing, treated this herb as a sacred plant. Wearing a wreath of bay leaves was a badge of honor for the triumphant ancient Greeks and Romans. Laurel leaves have been believed to protect people from the ancient deities that brought thunder and lightning.

The correlation between laurel leaves and glory has been relevant to modern times. We refer to completing a bachelor's degree as baccalaureate, which means "laurel berries." Hence, the idea of glory and honor are subsequently attached to the laurel leaves throughout history.

Habitat & Cultivation

Bay leaf is native to the region of the Mediterranean and has also been noted to grow very well in the woods of Europe, California, and Arab countries *(Spice Board India, n.d.).* These plants love to be cultivated in very sunny locations. For this reason, it grows well in the scorching climate of Arab countries.

It is a widespread garden herb that can be harvested year-round. The seeds take about nine months to germinate, and stem clippings take up to five months to root correctly. Be sure the soil drains well if you plan to grow this herb at home. If you plant it in a container, you can move it indoors if weather or temperature threatens growth.

Active Compounds: Up to 3% volatile oil consisting of 30–50% alpha-pinene, alpha-terpineol acetate, cineole, linalool, mucilage, tannin, and resin

Herbal Actions: Tonic effect; Stimulates appetite and secretion of digestive juices

Parts Used: Leaves and essential oil

Main Use:

- Ease arthritic aches and pains
- Upper digestive tract disorders
- Promotes digestion and absorption of food (breaks down heavy food, especially meat)

Self-care Use:

- Skin rashes
- Earaches
- Rheumatism (especially rheumatoid arthritis)
- Add a decoction of leaves to a bath to ease aches and pains in the limbs

⚠ **Caution!**

★ Bay leaf essential oil should NEVER be taken internally.

★ Allergic reactions may occur if applied externally. When making a bay leaf oil for external use, you should dilute your solution to a 2% concentration.

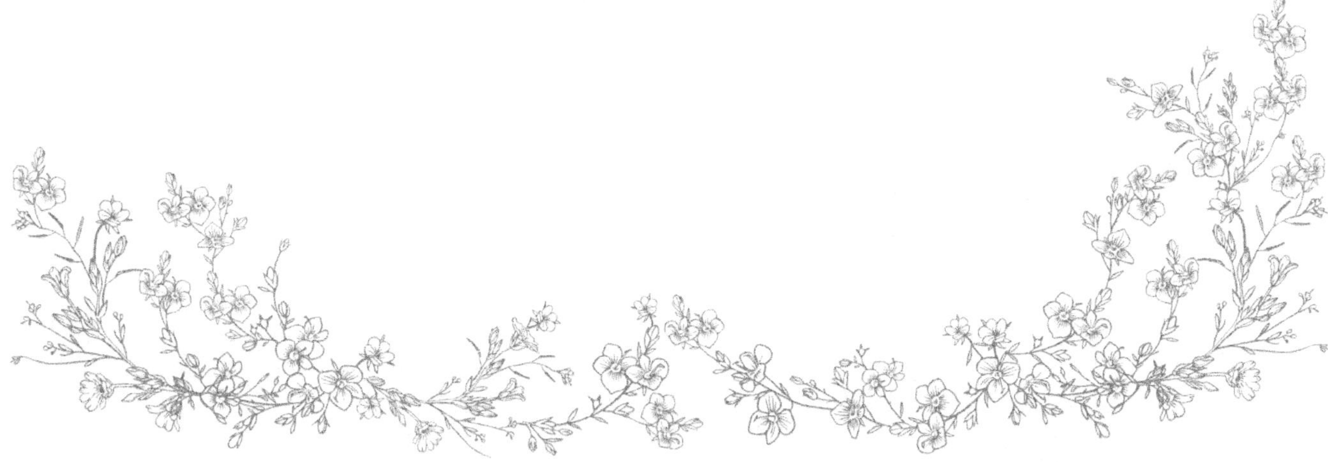

Chamomile

Chamomile recutita (Asteraceae)

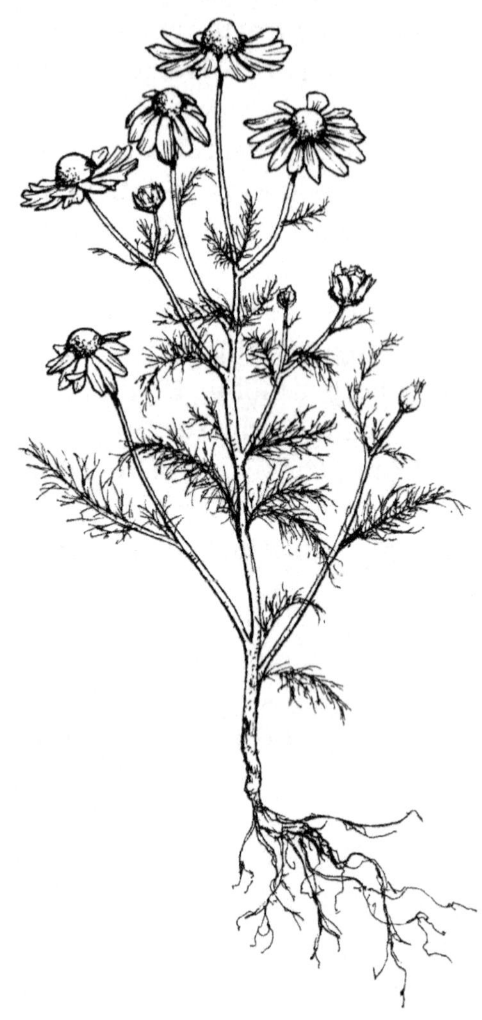

Chamomile has different preparations that cater to particular applications. Large quantities of terpenoids and flavonoids are extracted from dried chamomile flowers. Chamomile preparations help promote overall vitality as you can use them for common ailments like inflammation, fevers, wounds, pain, and much more *(Srivastava et al., 2010).* You can even utilize its essential oils for aromatherapy or steep tea for a relaxing warm drink to combat anxiety and upset stomachs.

I drink a cup of chamomile tea every night before bed. It is the one infusion that calms me down at the end of a hectic day. I suggest you add this to your self-care routine to unwind, release tension, and aid in a good night's rest.

Description

Chamomile is related to the daisy family and is a perennial plant that can grow between 8–21 inches (about 20.3–53.3 centimeters) tall. They have white petals, and the centers are composed of beautiful, brightly-colored gold cones. The appearance of this plant comes in tubular or disc-like florets that smell herbaceous, sweet, and somewhat apple-like.

History

Chamomile, as an herbal remedy, has a written history originating in Africa, Asia, and Europe. Because of this shrub's earthy and apple-like scent, the Greeks named it chamomile, meaning "earth apple." In Africa, the Egyptians revered this herb as a gift from the Sun God and used it in many ceremonies.

Hippocrates created an extensive list of the uses of chamomile during his time, including almost the same inventory we have for chamomile's herbal applications today *(Wong, 2021)*. Also, to further illustrate the impact of chamomile in history, the Germans refer to this plant as "alles zutraut," meaning "it can do anything!"

Habitat & Cultivation

Chamomile was originally native to Europe, Africa, and Asia but is now cultivated globally. You can see it growing freely in fields, pastures, and even along roadsides. Because of the versatility of this plant, you can easily add it to your herb garden. It is one of my favorite herbs to grow and use regularly.

While it might be easier to grow chamomile from its plant parts, do not let this discourage you from trying to grow it from seeds. Keeping your growing chamomile in a cool shade with dry soil can help it grow well. Chamomile can tolerate drought and naturally keeps unwanted pests away due to its strong smell. They tend to flower between May and October, depending on weather conditions.

Active Compounds: Volatile oil (proazulenes, farnesine, alpha-bisabolol, spiroether); Flavonoids; Bitter glycosides (anthemic acid); Cumbrians

Herbal Actions: Anti-inflammatory; Antispasmodic; Antiallergenic; Carminative; Relaxant

Parts Used: Flower heads (dried or fresh)

Main Use:

- Acidity, bolting, gas, gastritis, indigestion, pain, and colic
- Crohn's disease
- Peptic ulcers
- Irritable bowel syndrome
- Eases tense muscles and menstrual cramps
- Reduce irritability
- Promotes sleep
- Asthma and hay fever
- Externally used on sores and itchy skin (Eczema, sore nipples)

Self-care Use:

- Bites and stings
- Congestion
- Indigestion; Stomach spasms
- Insomnia
- Morning sickness
- Mild asthma

⚠ **Caution!**

★ DO NOT use essential oil externally during PREGNANCY
★ DO NOT use essential oil internally (only under doctor supervision)
★ Check with your doctor first if you are on blood-thinning medication
★ Fresh plant can cause dermatitis

Catnip

Nepeta catarina (Lamiaceae)

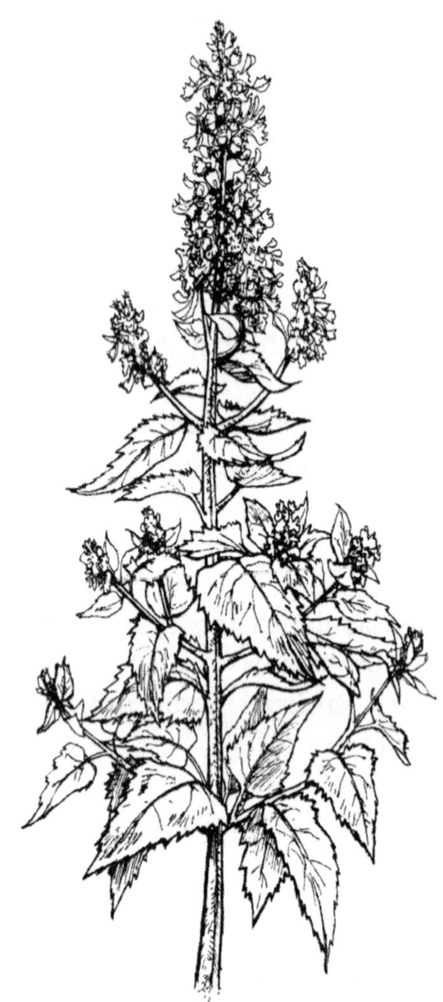

Catnip is an herb famous for being used in toys for cats. However, it can provide a calming effect for people, which helps provide better vitality *(Cronkleton, 2021)*. While there are various ways to use catnip, the best-known form to take advantage of its relaxing benefits is to brew it as tea. In addition to tea, you can also make tinctures or decoctions.

I recall having lunch with a friend that suffered from multiple panic attacks. She worked at a big marketing firm and often presented big deals to multi-billion dollar companies. My friend took synthetic anxiety medication but was worried about the side effects she encountered. That is when I introduced her to catnip. She now takes catnip infusions, tinctures, or supplements when she starts to feel panicky or nervous before a big presentation.

Description

Catnip is a mint family member and short-lived perennial that grows between 2–3 feet (about 61–91 centimeters) tall. The plants have heart-shaped leaves with toothed edges that are light, dark, or grayish-green colored. The leaves and stems are covered in fuzzy hairs and typically accompanied by white flowers. These characteristics are similar to other plants within the mint family, but catnip has a lighter minty sage-like smell.

History

Catnip, or Nepeta catarina, is believed to have its name from "Nepete" and "cataria." Nepete was a town in Italy, while "cataria" is the Latin word that refers to cats. There is not much known about the early applications of catnip. Still, it has been documented that some Northeastern Native Americans used it as an aid for easing upset stomachs and sleeplessness.

We know of its documentation during the 1730s in a book called "General Irish Herbal," where catnip leaves and flowers were steeped in tea and used for different herbal purposes *(drugs.com, n.d.).* Furthermore, in the 1960s, people smoked dried leaves to take advantage of their euphoric properties.

Habitat & Cultivation

Catnip is an herb native to Central Europe but now grows in most parts of Canada and the Northeast United States. Although catnip is not the type of plant that gets picky with its soil and growing location, it prefers well-draining soil. It loves to have full sunlight, grows fast, and blooms between spring and autumn *(James, 2016).* It is also not that difficult to find yourself a catnip plant as you forage.

Active Compounds: Iridoids; Tannins; Volatile oil (alpha-nepetalactone, beta-nepetalactone, citronellol, and geraniol)

Herbal Actions: Sedative; Stimulates sweating; Antiflatulent

Parts Used: Aerial parts

Main Use:

- Helps reduce fever by encouraging sweating
- Colds, flus, and fever in children
- Calming effect for the body

Self-care Use:

- Digestive infections: Settles the stomach and helps with indigestion
- Headaches related to digestive issues
- Tincture used for rheumatism and arthritis (rub vigorously over affected area)

⚠ Caution!

- ★ Excessive drowsiness when used alongside other sedative medication
- ★ In large quantities may cause vomiting, headaches, and lethargy
- ★ Can lead to dehydration if taken in massive amounts

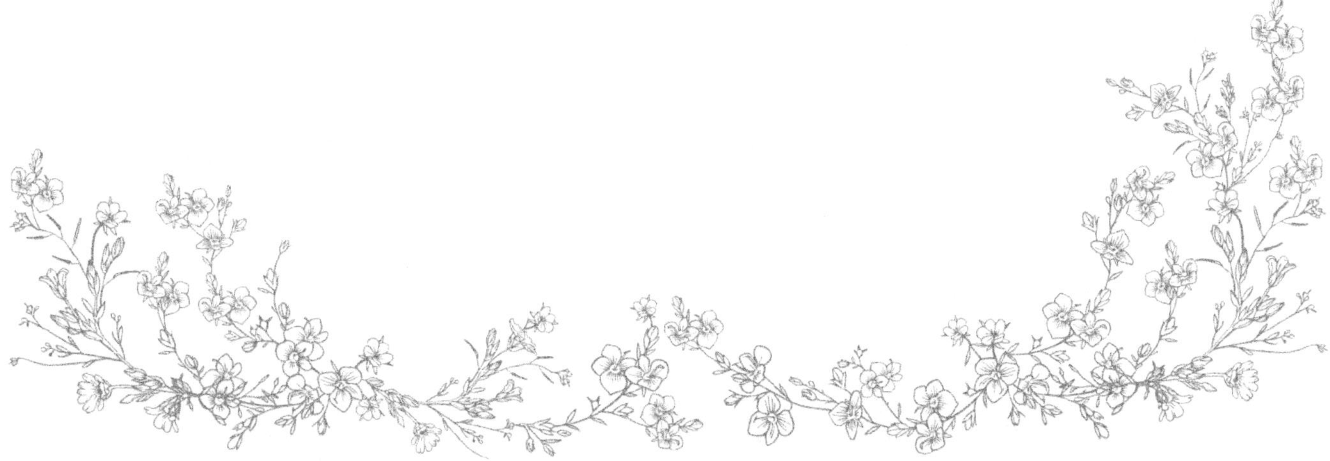

Cayenne Pepper

Capsicum annuum (Solanaceae)

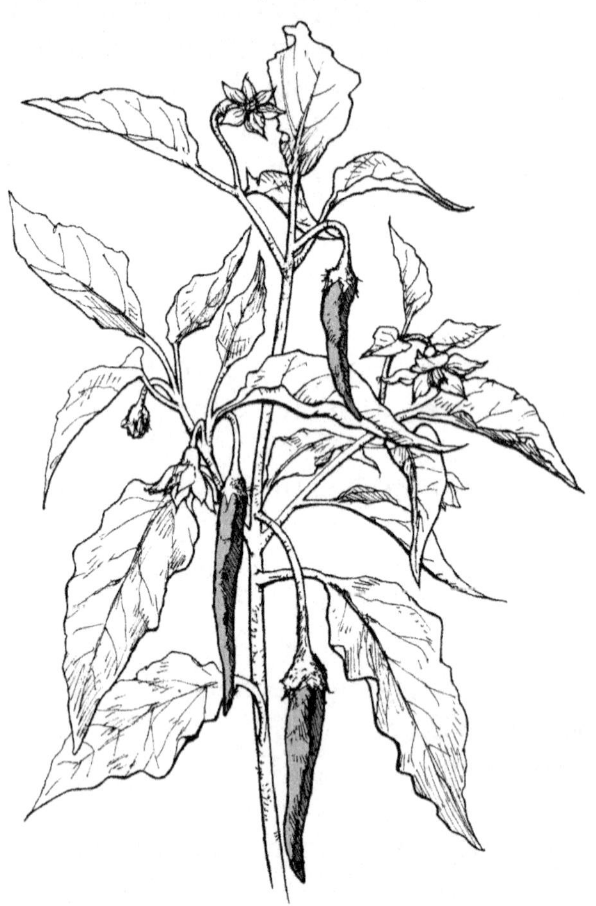

Cayenne pepper is typically used in dishes that need an extra spicy kick! The capsaicin content gives that mouth-tingling spice flavor. It produces high levels of vitamins A, B6, E, and C and minerals like potassium and manganese *(Grant, 2021)*. Aside from the spice that cayenne peppers have, they also have numerous benefits for optimizing your vitality.

These peppers can boost your metabolism, reduce your appetite, effectively reduce blood pressure, and much more *(Raman, 2017)*. Most of the benefits of cayenne peppers come from the capsaicin content. Cayenne pepper is one of my go-to recommendations if you have a cold. This spice is excellent for congestion, postnasal drip, sneezing, and stuffy noses.

Description

The appearance of the cayenne pepper is glossy and narrow, with a curved tip and rippled skin. The fruit is typically red when ripe, although green or yellow is often picked. This pepper is mild and grows in lengths of about 4–10 inches (about 10–25 centimeters) long on the bushy cayenne plant.

History

The cayenne peppers' name comes from the city of Cayenne, in South America, where these peppers are known to originate. During ancient times Native Americans were already utilizing cayenne peppers for food and herbal use, especially for stomach aches and circulatory problems *(Encyclopedia, 2018)*. As the era of exploration began, Christopher Columbus aided in bringing cayenne peppers to Europe. Eventually, transportation took this plant to tropical countries where it grows best.

Habitat & Cultivation

The spicy cayenne peppers need to grow in relatively hot areas. They thrive well in tropical and subtropical regions with a lot of sunlight. However, these plants can be sensitive to too hot or cold environments. Cayenne pepper plants need around 100–120 days before they mature. Growing cayenne peppers well requires moderate water and moist, fertile soils. They grow as perennials in their native hot habitats but can be cultivated annually in temperate climates.

Active Compounds: Capsaicin (0.1–1.5%) only in the seeds; Carotenoids; Flavonoids; Steroidal saponins; Volatile oil

Herbal Actions: Analgesic; Antimicrobial; Antiseptic; Carminative; Relieves muscle spasms; Stimulant; Tonic

Parts Used: Fresh and dried fruit

Main Use:

- Capsaicin applied to the skin may help with neurological pain by desensitizing nerve endings
- Possible pain relief: arthritis and headaches
- Antimicrobial: intestinal or gastric infections; Gastroenteritis and dysentery
- Stimulant: improves circulation

Self-care Use:

- High fever
- Poor circulation
- Relieves gas
- Sore throats
- Relieves acute diarrhea

⚠ **Caution!**

★ HOT! Can cause burning, pain, and contact dermatitis
★ Non-toxic in low doses, but caution should be taken when eating or handling!
★ Eating too much in one meal can lead to an upset stomach.

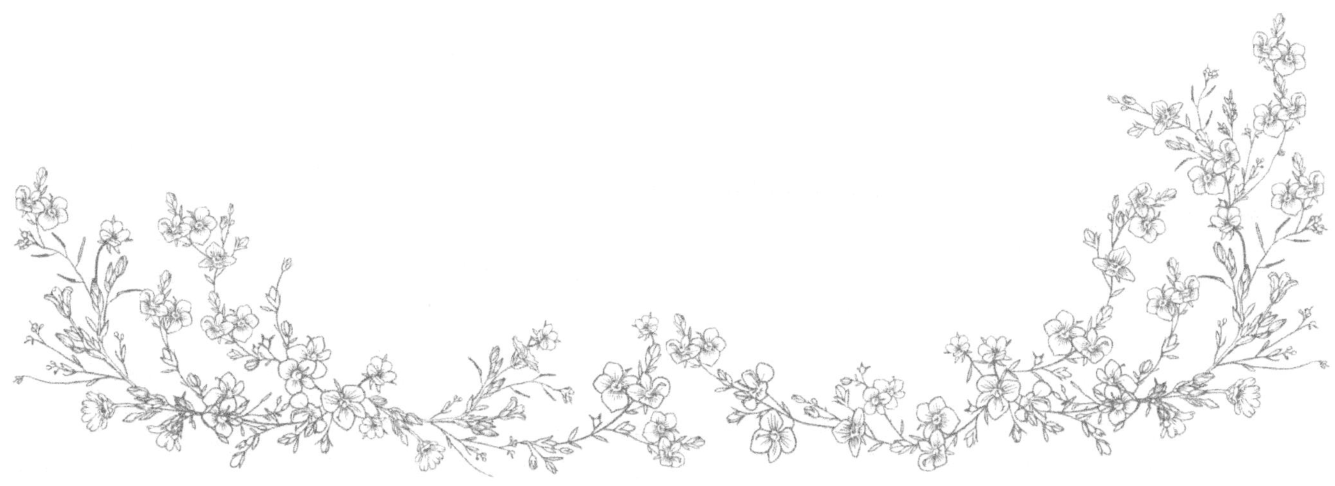

Cinnamon

Cinnamomum verum (Lauraceae)

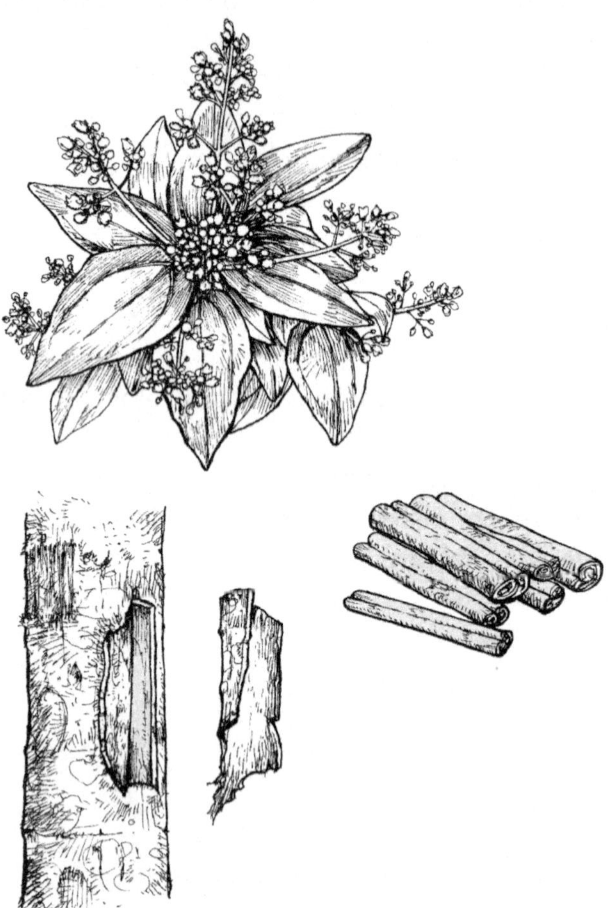

Cinnamon gives a unique savory taste and aroma that is fit for being a common household spice. The sticks you can purchase come from peeling and drying bark from a cinnamon tree. You can also spot this spice sold in powder form as it is commonly used in baking. Cinnamon has also been linked to many health benefits, including controlling blood sugar and aiding in inflammatory responses.

I utilize a tablespoon in my daily protein shake for an extra boost of flavor and to help keep inflammation at bay. If you are like me and live with a chronic inflammatory condition, you should add cinnamon to your daily diet and see if it helps.

Description

The cinnamon tree is a bushy evergreen plant that can grow 4–5 feet (1.22–1.52 meters) tall indoors and about 20–30 feet (6.1–9.14 meters) or higher outdoors. The inner bark is dried to become the aromatic spice we all know. This spice tastes warm and sweet, and the pungent smell and taste come from a chemical compound known as cinnamaldehyde. When first cultivated, it is a golden-yellow color and darkens as it ages, forming resinous compounds.

History

Deriving from the Hebraic and Arabic term "amomon," meaning fragrant spice plant, this botanical has been used for centuries. The Egyptians used it in their embalming practices, and the monks during the Middle Ages utilized it for sore throats, coughing, and hoarseness. They also often used cinnamon to preserve or mask the smell of spoiling meat *(Filippone, 2019)*. Cinnamon continued to grow in population, and by 1833 the plant started to be cultivated worldwide.

Habitat & Cultivation

Cinnamon is native to Sri Lanka (formerly Ceylon) and India and grows at an altitude of around 1,600–3,281 feet (500–1000 meters) in tropical forests. It is also found in the Caribbean and Philippine islands. In India, crops are rain-reliant on an annual rainfall of approximately 6.5–8.2 feet (200–250 centimeters) and can be grown in low nutrient-rich soil *(Suvidha, 2017)*. When the trees reach about two years old, they are cut back to ground level and covered with dirt. This technique, done every year, makes the trees grow like a bush, and the plant will produce new branches the following year. When harvested, the shoots are stripped, and the bark is set out to dry in the sun. The sun-dried strips will naturally curl and form the iconic quill sticks.

Active Compounds: Volatile oil up to 4% (cinnamaldehyde 65–80%, eugenol 5–10%); Phenolics (procyanidins); Mucilage

Herbal Actions: Antidiabetic; Antimicrobial; Anti-inflammatory; Antifungal; Carminative; Warming stimulant

Parts Used: Inner bark and twigs

Main Use:

- Type 2 diabetes
- Strong antioxidant
- Stimulates blood flow to the extremities
- Digestive issues
- Loss of appetite

Self-care Use:

- Cold and flu-like symptoms
- Bronchitis
- Mouthwash for oral thrush

⚠ **Caution!**

- ★ Occasional allergic reactions
- ★ Excessive use may cause low blood sugar
- ★ DO NOT take essential oil internally (external use only!)

Clove

Eugenia caryophyllata (Myrtaceae)

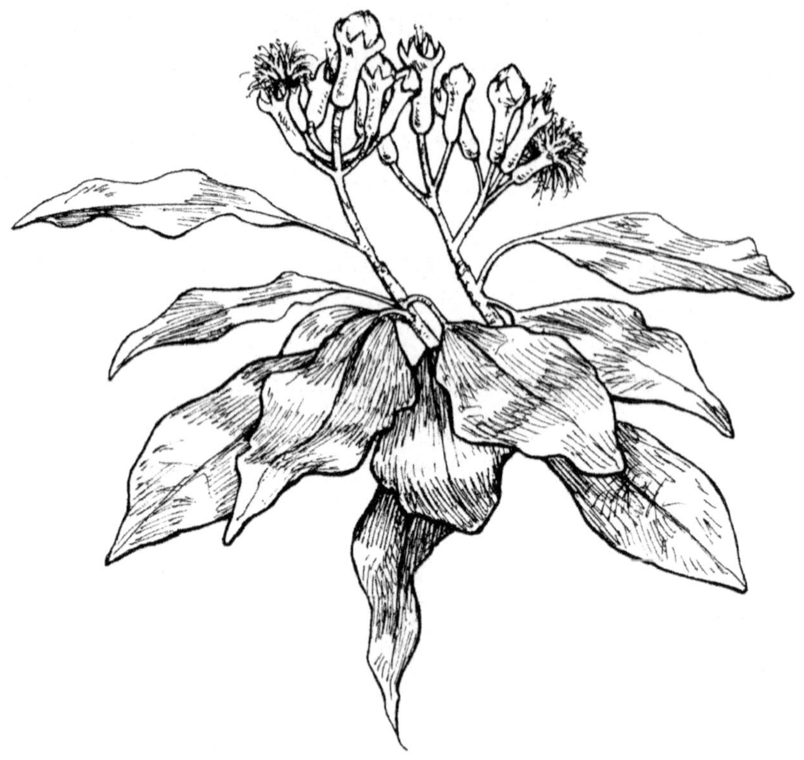

In many regions, clove has broad uses in food preparation as it gives a strong aromatic scent and a slight tingling sensation on the tongue *(Singh et al., 2012).* Of course, cloves also have traditional medicinal uses that have been around for centuries. These plants have active components that can promote better stomach health, reduce inflammation, temporarily aid toothaches, and help decongest clogged sinuses. The versatility of cloves makes it possible for them to be utilized by pharmaceutical companies and the perfume and cosmetic industries.

Clove oil was one of the first herbal remedies I was introduced to as a child. My mom consistently applied it to my gum line for its numbing effects whenever I had a toothache. I still utilize it for tooth pain to this day!

Description

The clove plant is an aromatic evergreen tree that can grow 25–40 feet (8–12 meters) tall. This tree sprouts pale-colored flower buds that become a green to dark brown or dusky red color. Its bark is gray, and its leaves resemble bay leaves at around 5 inches (13 centimeters) long. Essential oils can be extracted from the clove's dried flower buds, and the aromatic scent extracted from the oils holds the vital compounds.

History

Cloves were found in Syria in ceramic vessels as far back as 1721 BC. It was one of the first spices traded outside of its native region. Initially, the Dutch monopolized cloves during the age of exploration (17th century). In the late 18th century, the French smuggled these plants out of the East Indies to the Indian Ocean and New World.

Ayurvedic medicine, Chinese medicine, and even the Western world used cloves for their medicinal properties. Some believed that cloves could alleviate problems with parasites like tapeworms and roundworms, help with dental concerns like toothaches and sore throat, and even help with respiratory and digestive troubles *(Singh et al., 2012).* Clove's fascinating history paved the way for modern medicinal plant research being executed today.

Habitat & Cultivation

The Maluku Islands of Indonesia are the home of native clove trees *(Singh et al., 2012).* The plant eventually gained a place as a spice cultivated around the world. Indonesia has a warm and humid tropical climate that makes cloves thrive. The land must have rich and loamy soils with good drainage to ensure a clove tree grows well. It takes about six years for the tree to produce viable flowers and 20 years to fully mature.

A mature tree can produce fruit for nearly 80 years! Buds will mature at different times and are gathered from the same tree every other year. Once the buds are harvested, they are laid out in the sun on tarps to dry. The buds will turn from green to reddish-brown as they dry. The extracts of these dried plant parts give us beneficial active compounds.

Active Compounds: Tannins; Gum; Volatile oil eugenol (approximately 85%), acetyl eugenol, methyl salicylate, pinene, vanillin

Herbal Actions: Analgesic; Antimicrobial; Antiseptic; Antispasmodic; Carminative; Eliminates parasites; Prevents vomiting; Stimulant

Parts Used: Flower buds (usually dried); Leaves and stems (oil extraction)

Main Use:

- All-purpose remedy
- Antiseptic: Viral conditions (ex: malaria, cholera, and tuberculosis); Parasites (scabies)
- Digestive issues: gas, bolting, and colic
- Eases coughs
- Topically relieves muscle spasms
- Improves memory
- Aphrodisiac
- Preparation for childbirth (strengthens and stimulates contractions during labor)

Self-care Use:

- Acne and boils
- Fever
- Fungal skin infections
- Neuralgia
- Toothaches

⚠ **Caution!**

- ★ DO NOT use essential oil internally (only under doctor supervision)
- ★ Dermatitis may occur with external use

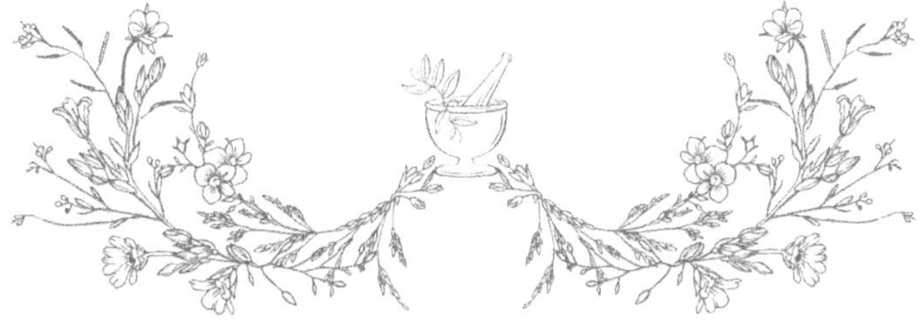

Eleuthero

Eleutherococcus senticosus (Araliaceae)

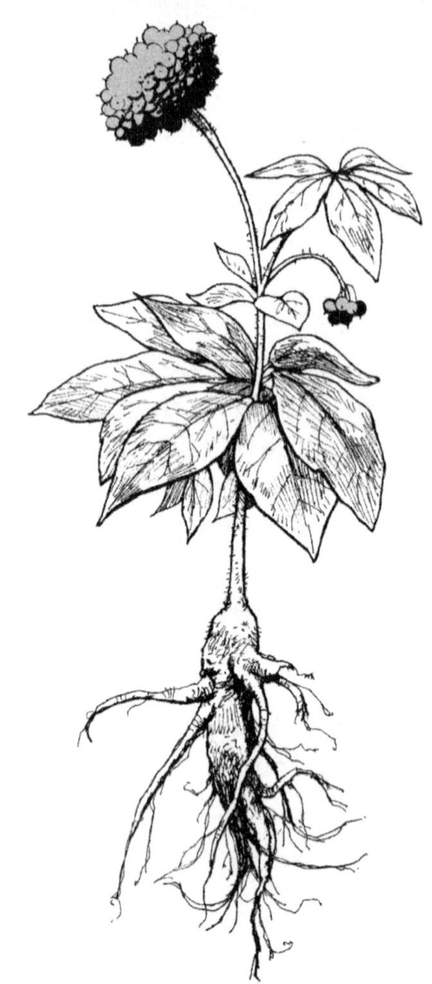

Eleuthero is an adaptogen and stimulant that may help improve your cognitive function by optimizing blood flow to your brain *(Huizen, 2017).* The dried leaves and stems can be brewed to make tea, while the fruits can be taken raw to maximize the active components and nutrients.

I utilize eleuthero powders in my workout shakes to help with endurance. I have even recommended it to others in the gym. I always get rave reviews! The recommended daily dose is 3-6 grams; even though it does not raise your estrogen levels, it still binds to your estrogen receptors. Only take eleuthero powder for six weeks and then take a two to three-week break.

Description

Eleuthero is a small woody shrub that, when consumed, has a sharp and slightly bitter taste. Typically the plant grows 2–3 feet (about 61–91.4 centimeters) tall, but it can grow as tall as 20 feet (6.1 meters) if space permits. This herb is sometimes called Siberian ginseng, but it must not be confused with American or Panax ginseng. All of these herbs look similar when compared side by side. The similarity in appearance is not translated to their chemical and herbal applications, as their effects are entirely different. Using "eleuthero" as the designated name will alleviate the confusion with American or Panax ginseng.

History

China held one of the first pieces of evidence of eleuthero's herbal applications and was noted as far back as 2000 years ago *(Huizen, 2017).* In Traditional Chinese Medicine, eleuthero was and is still referred to as "ci wu jia," meaning "many-prickle."

Eleuthero's confusion with other ginseng herbs began as they used to be grouped under the same Panax family due to their adaptogenic effects *(Fidler, 2017).* Research and development concluded that the significant difference was in the content of one vital active compound. The ginsenosides found in American and Panax ginseng were not found in eleuthero; hence, they do not belong in the same group.

Habitat & Cultivation

Eleuthero is native to several regions in Asia, including Japan, Northern China, Southeastern Russia, and Korea. This plant grows at a relatively slow pace. To ensure your eleuthero grows at a healthy rate, you should plant them 6–10 feet (2–3 meters) apart from each other. This plant thrives in full sunlight and moist soil in northern regions. When residing in warmer southern areas, you will want to plant this herb in the shade and keep the soil nice and wet. The rhizomes mature and are harvested around four to five years after planting.

Active Compounds: Eleutherosides (0.6-0.9%); Glycans; Polysaccharides; Triterpenoid saponins

Herbal Actions: Adaptogenic; Protects the immune system; Tonic; Stimulant stamina and resistance to stress

Parts Used: Root (dried or fresh)

Main Use:

- Stamina for athletic performance: reduces stress on the body
- Cancer treatment: promotes vitality in chemotherapy patients
- Improves mental resilience
- Helps with chronic fatigue

Self-care Use:

- Convalescence
- Menopause
- Stress

⚠ **Caution!**

★ DO NOT use for a long time unless under the supervision of a doctor
★ Healthy young people should not take longer than 6 weeks
★ Rare side effects when taken as directed in a standard dose for short periods of time
★ Avoid caffeine in conjunction with eleuthero

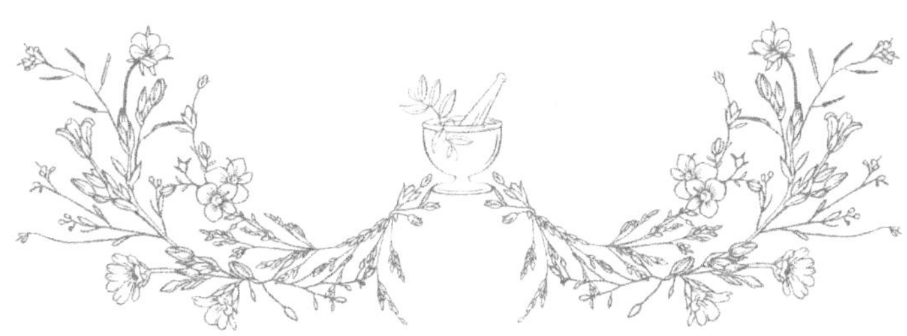

Frankincense (Olibanum)

Boswellia serrata (Burseraceae)

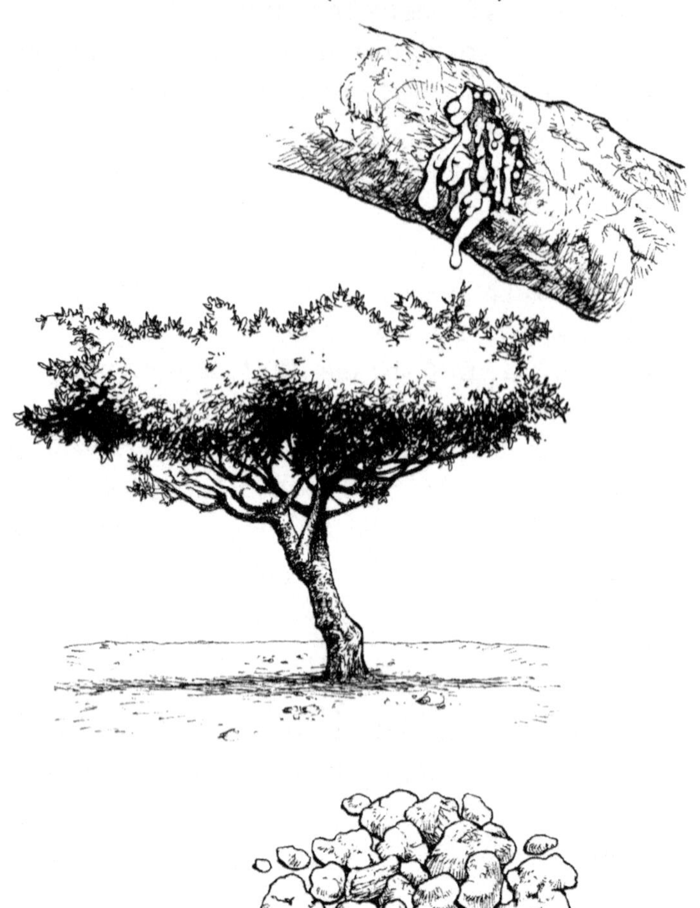

Some ways to use frankincense are to inhale its essence, absorb it on the skin, or take it as an oral supplement. This plant has varied benefits, from aiding digestion, asthma-alleviation, and maintaining oral health *(Petre, 2021)*. Known as the "king of essential oils," it has versatile all-natural aromatherapy benefits with minimal side effects *(Levenberg, 2020)*. Frankincense oil has concentrated active compounds and should be diluted before use in most herbal remedies.

Frankincense is hands down my favorite essential oil. If I have had an overly stressful day, I make myself a nice cup of tea and draw myself a bath. I put 10 or 12 drops of frankincense oil in my Epsom salt bath for additional relaxing effects.

Description

Frankincense has a woody body with a spicy odor. This essential oil is extracted from the inner bark of trees. While the trees resemble bonsai trees, they grow much taller at around 6–26 feet (2–8 meters) tall. They can have one or two trunks with paper-like bark. The outer bark is removed with ease to get to the inner layer.

History

Frankincense is chiefly utilized for its essential oils. Historically, this oil was one of the gifts presented on the night of Jesus' birth. Ancient religious societies used frankincense oil to symbolize power. They also anointed people with the oil and used it in prayers and rituals *(Levenberg, 2020)*. Frankincense is a unique commodity that has been traded for thousands of years.

Habitat & Cultivation

This tree typically grows in India, the Middle East, and Africa, as these places have vast mountainous regions with dry climates. There has been a very high demand for aromatic oils and resins from the frankincense tree. For this reason, it has been near extinction since about 1998 and has yet to regenerate *(Fobar, 2019)*. Other causes include wildfires, insect infestation, animal grazing, and improper harvesting.

Active Compounds: Essential oil; Monosaccharides; Tannins; Triterpene acids (beta-boswellic acid); Sterols; Uronic acids

Herbal Actions: Anti-inflammatory; Antiarthritic; Antiseptic; Astringent

Parts Used: Gum resin, bark

Main Use:

- Inflammatory bowel disease
- Psoriasis
- Ulcerative colitis
- Rheumatoid arthritis
- Helps tighten inflamed mucous membranes
- Canker sores
- Sore throat
- Laryngitis
- Gum disease
- Stabilizes blood glucose in people who have type 2 diabetes

Self-care Use:

- Asthma and hay fever
- Pain reliever

⚠ **Caution!**

- ★ External use of essential oil may cause dermatitis
- ★ Internal use of extract is possibly safe in 100 milligram doses up to 6 months, usually with no side effects. Some may experience heartburn, itching, nausea, diarrhea, and stomach pains.

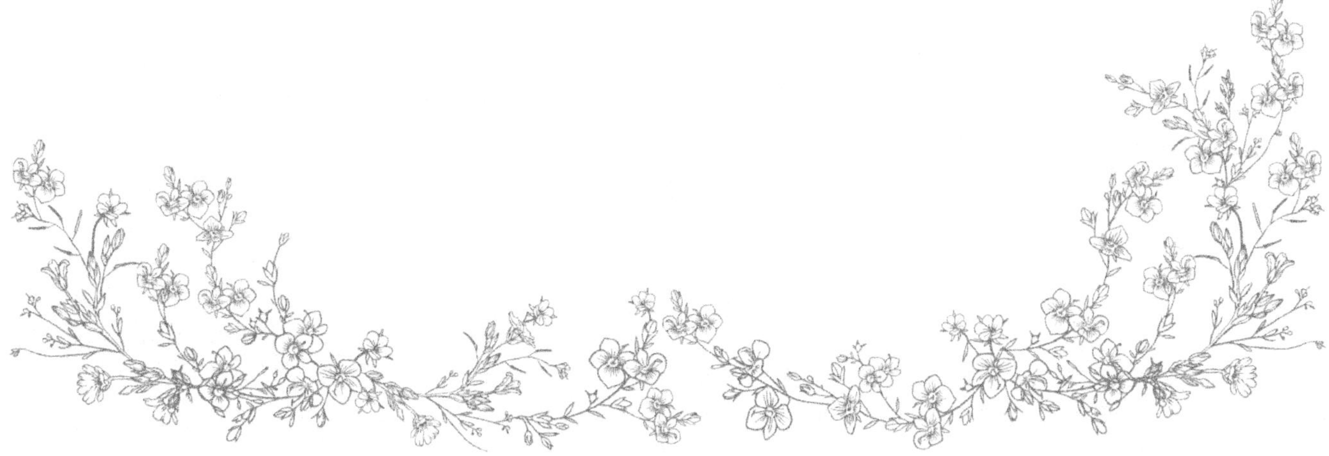

Ginger

Zingiber officinale (Zingiberaceae)

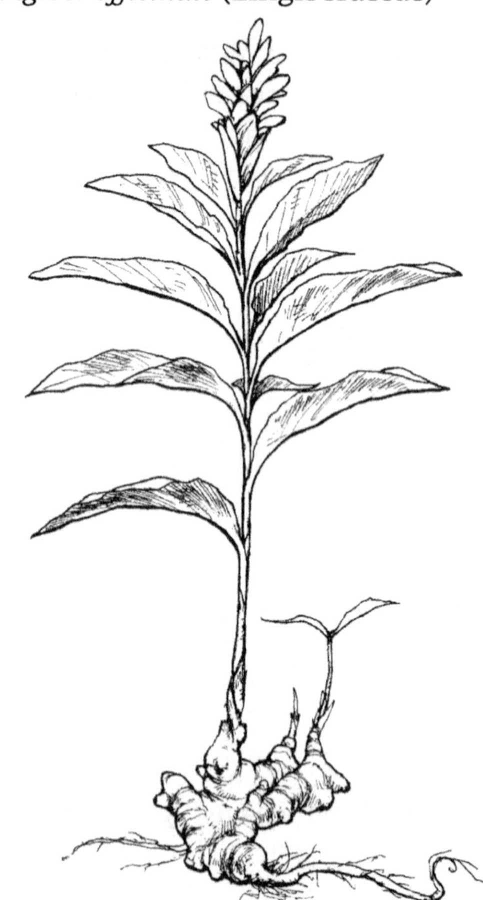

Adding thinly sliced or grated ginger imparts a robust flavor to dishes, but the wonders of ginger are not limited to its rich flavor. Ginger supports health conditions such as common colds, hypertension, nausea, arthritis, migraines, and much more *(Benzie & Wachtel-Galor, 2011)*. Add it to a cup of tea to strengthen your immune system.

I use ginger infusions regularly to maintain my overall wellness and increase my dosage if I have a belly ache or indigestion. It keeps my immune system running at its highest capacity. I believe ginger is probably one of the main reasons I rarely get sick.

Description

Ginger rhizomes hold the majority of the active compounds found in this plant. It grows relatively close to the soil's surface with knots that often pop through the soil line. The ginger plants' aerial parts have reed-like stalks that grow to about 3 feet (1 meter) tall and are topped with yellow flowers. The aroma is slightly spicy and citrusy but has woody and floral notes as well. The taste is described as spicy and pepper-like with an intense feel.

History

Ginger is part of a plant family related to cardamom and turmeric. Over 3000 years ago, the Sanskrit word "srngaveram," meaning "horn body," was the initial name of this spice. However, the Middle English term "gingivere" gave the current name to ginger *(Benzie & Wachtel-Galor, 2011)*. The richness of ginger and its medicinal usage is mentioned in India, China, Greece, and the Mediterranean's histories.

Ginger was openly traded over 2000 years ago and was even taxed by the Roman Empire. This spice was lost to most of Europe when the Roman Empire fell. It reappeared during the 11th century when Marco Polo brought it back from one of his many explorations. Today it continues to be a desirable spice and has value in traditional and modern medications.

Habitat & Cultivation

India is the largest cultivator of ginger because of this region's humid and tropical weather. Africa and South America also have the appropriate climate for the commercial production of this spice. Moist and fertile soil is best, and some people add a layer of peat moss to keep the soil adequately damp.

If cultivating at home, you can put your young ginger plants in the ground after the first frost has passed in the spring. It will take about 8–10 months for the plant to mature, and you should harvest it in the first part of winter as the leaves begin to wilt. Choose a good root from your harvest to cultivate the following year.

Active Compounds: Volatile oil (1–3%); Zingiberene (20–30%); Oleoresins (4–7.5%); Gingerol and shogaols

Herbal Actions: Antiemetic; Anti-inflammatory; Antiviral; Circulatory and Digestive stimulant

Parts Used: Rhizome (dried or fresh)

Main Use:

- Pain relief
- Digestive health
- Circulation
- Respiratory conditions

Self-care Use:

- Cold, flu, and fever
- Cold sores
- Constipation
- Colic, digestive upset, and gas
- High blood pressure
- Morning sickness
- Motion sickness and nausea

⚠ Caution!

★ DO NOT use essential oil internally (only under doctor supervision)

★ DO NOT take if you have peptic ulcers

★ If you are taking anticoagulants or if you are PREGNANT the recommended daily dose is no more than 4 grams fresh root (2 grams dried).

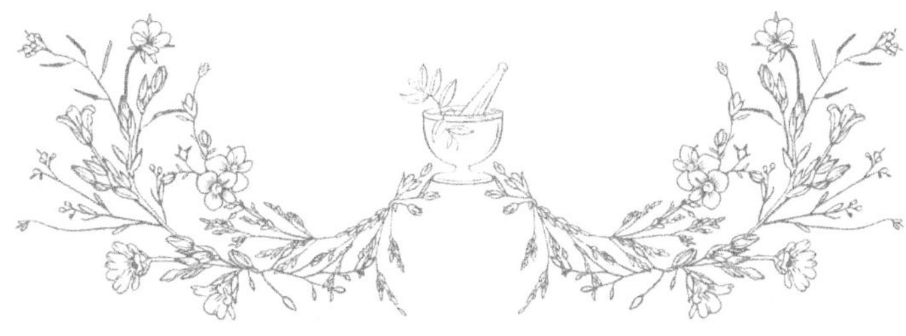

Ginseng (American)

Panax quinquefolius (Araliaceae)

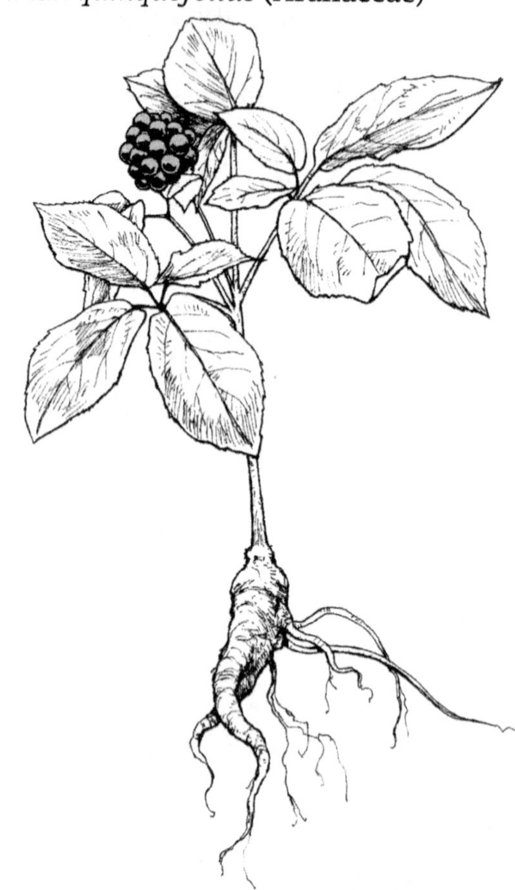

American ginseng has been part of Traditional Native American medicine for thousands of years. American and Korean ginsengs have benefits that include reducing inflammatory markers, protecting from oxidative stress, improving brain capacity, and boosting the immune system *(Semeco, 2018)*. American ginseng is available in various forms, including powders, capsules, or tablets.

A ginseng decoction was first recommended to me when I had some gastrointestinal issues. It made me feel rejuvenated and healthier than I had felt in years. My stress levels were lowered, and my inflamed gut nearly disappeared overnight.

Description

American ginseng root is a light tan and is gnarled in appearance – often resembles human bodies as its shoots can be imagined as arms and legs. The stalk is relatively long, sprouting to about 1–2 feet (30.5–61 centimeters) tall adorning ovate-shaped leaves. Although ginseng root tastes primarily bitter, it also has notes of woody sweetness. The berries are bright red with a somewhat tart taste but are also safe to eat. Try not to confuse American with Korean Panax ginseng. They may have similar appearances, but the plants are entirely different species.

History

Based on the plant's name, its history is traced back to North America. The Native Americans have been taking advantage of the stimulating effects of this herb for centuries. They used, and still use, it to help with health issues like headaches, infertility, or fever. European colonizers in the early 1700s also appreciated the value of this herb and applied it to their own needs. Today,

American ginseng can fetch a trade cost of as much as $600 a pound with overseas countries, especially in East Asia.

Habitat & Cultivation

American ginseng thrives well in the eastern deciduous forests of North America. It can take up to eight years to reach maturity and be ready for harvesting. This maturity happens ***before*** clusters of flowers or umbels are produced.

If you want to grow this herb at home, choose an area that drains well and ensure the soil is dark with high calcium and organic matter content. Throw a healthy layer of leaf mulch on top. The little sprouts are hard to see, but your ginseng will be ready to harvest within a few short years.

Active Compounds: Triterpenoid saponins (0.07–3%); Ginsenosides (25 identified); Gintonin; Acetylenic; Panaxans; Sesquiterpenes

Herbal Actions: Adaptogen; Anti-inflammatory; Tonic

Parts Used: Root (dried or fresh)

Main Use:

- Adapt to colds and fatigue
- Mental and emotional stress
- Cope with hunger
- Helps the body adapt to extreme temperatures
- Hormonal support: Deficient hormonal states (ginsenosides have similar structures to hormones found in the body).

Self-care Use:

- Impotence and premature ejaculation
- Menopausal symptoms (hot flashes, lowered mood, and improves sexual arousal)
- Maintaining vitality
- Poor sleep and exhaustion
- Short-term stress

⚠ **Caution!**

★ DO NOT use if PREGNANT
★ Avoid caffeine in conjunction with ginseng
★ May interfere with depression medications (check with your doctor)
★ Healthy young people should not take longer than 6 weeks
★ DO NOT exceed the recommended dose. Taking more may cause high blood pressure and insomnia. (Daily dosage: 1–2 grams of dried powder, 0.5–3 grams raw root, or 100–800 milligrams extract)

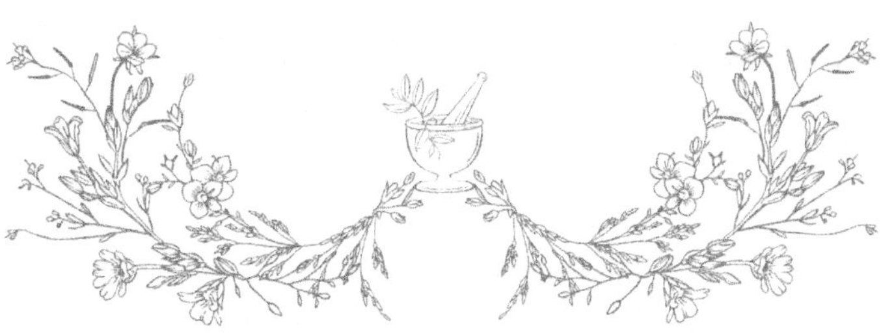

Green Tea

Camellia sinensis (Theaceae)

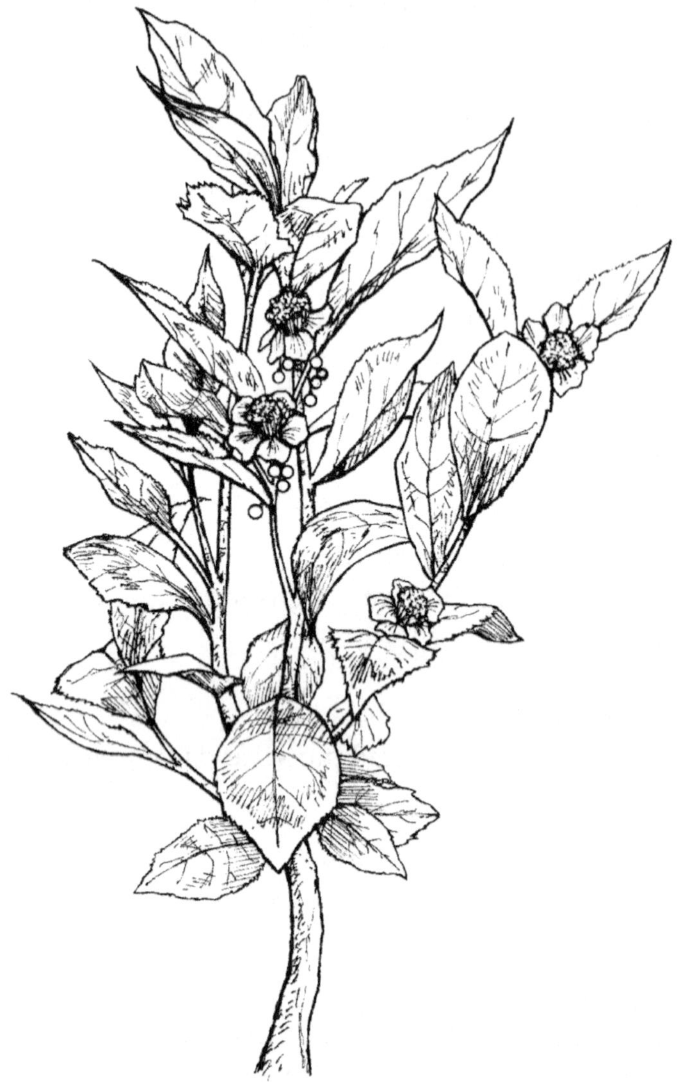

Camellia sinensis is a plant that can be steeped as Green, Black, or Oolong tea. Despite the differences, they generally produce the same health benefits due to the active components extracted from them. Green tea is made by immediately steaming the freshly harvested leaves to ensure that essential enzymes remain in the tea after brewing in the comfort of your home.

I love a good infusion of green tea, but I also like to take a little green tea extract after a workout. A trainer friend recommended it to me when I started going back to the gym. I had not lifted weights since high school and felt like I was going to die after each training session. Then I started putting a little green tea extract in my post-workout shake. I noticed that the recovery time after training sessions was significantly less. This extract is my number one suggestion to anyone who works out regularly. Plus, it also promotes weight loss!

Description

Although there are many types of tea, the green tea plant is a perennial tree or shrub. Well-kept plants are generally cut back to about 3–5 feet (1–1.5 meters) tall. Leaves are dark green, spear-shaped, and come to a point. They grow to about 2–3 inches (5–7.6 centimeters) long, usually have fuzz on the underside, and feel somewhat leathery.

History

Green tea originated in China as far back as 2737 BC, when Chinese Emperor Shennong accidentally discovered it. Initially, green tea was only available to the elite of society. It was eventually accepted as a new beverage to quench thirst. In the 14th century, it became accessible to the general public as a refreshing drink and an herbal remedy.

Green tea was also used in Traditional Chinese Medicine and Indian practices to manage excess bleeding and heal wounds. Aside from these, today, other herbal benefits include using green tea to support digestion, heart, and mental health *(Ware, 2021)*. Green tea extract can now be found in over-the-counter forms like powders, tablets, capsules, and liquids.

Habitat & Cultivation

Tea is an essential drink all around the globe. Its cultivation is very commercialized as an estimated 2.5 million tons of dried tea leaves are annually made worldwide *(Chaco et al., 2010)*. China's rich history with green tea makes it the most prominent place to produce it.

The tea plant thrives in its natural habitat of tropical and subtropical forests. If you want to grow this herb at home, you can propagate it outside if you live in a warm climate or indoors if you are in a cooler area. You can buy a start from a nursery, use a clipping, or start from seed. The seeds take about four weeks to germinate, and it can take up to three years before you can harvest the leaves for tea.

Active Compounds: Caffeine (1-5%); Flavonoids; Fats; Vitamin C; Tannins (especially high amounts of polyphenols)

Herbal Actions: Antioxidant; Anti-inflammatory; Antibacterial; Astringent; Nerve tonic

Parts Used: Flower buds and leaves

Main Use:

- Polyphenols may help prevent cancer
- Slows the aging process
- Digestive infections
- Insect stings, swelling, sunburns, and minor burns
- Headaches (caffeine)

Self-care Use:

- Promote weight loss
- Helps prevent tooth decay

⚠ Caution!

★ DO NOT drink more than 8 cups of green tea a day. Doing so may cause irregular heartbeat and induce headaches.

★ DO NOT take green tea if you are PREGNANT or plan to become pregnant.

★ DO NOT take green tea extract on an empty stomach.

★ Green tea extract in high doses may cause liver injuries or failure.

Hemp Seed Oil

Cannabis sativa (Cannabaceae); Seeds

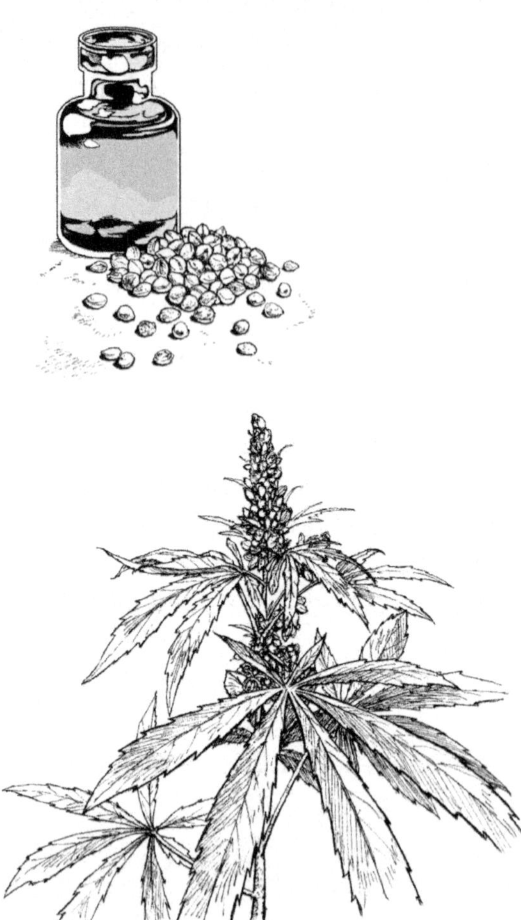

Hemp is closely related to the different variations of the Cannabis plant. However, hemp seed oil does not have the euphoric and psychotropic action you usually think of when talking about Cannabis. Science does not differentiate between the hemp plant and the marijuana plant. The significant difference between the two is the tetrahydrocannabinol (THC) content.

Hemp has significantly lower levels of THC. In contrast, you get a beneficial amount of omega-3 and omega-6 fatty acids, which keep your heart and vessels healthy *(Rodriguez-Leyva & Pierce, 2010)*. The rich fatty acids in hemp seed oils also keep the skin healthy and protect it from inflammation and early aging *(Johnson, 2019)*. Hemp seed oil uses the plants' seeds instead of the stalks or leaves known to have the "euphoric" compounds in Cannabis plants.

Are you stressed out and need an alternative to herbal teas and tinctures? I suggest trying hemp seed oil supplements regularly. It takes about 2–3 months to see the effects of this fantastic oil, but once you start taking it, I can assure you it will change your world.

Description

Cannabis sativa plants are dioecious, meaning separate male and female plants. The plant can reach an extraordinary height of about 25–35 feet (7.6–10.7 meters), depending on the growth space. They have slender stalks that are hollow except at the base and tip. The leaves are described as either palmate-shaped or sessile leaflets. Its seed-bearing flowers can be observed growing in small spike-like clusters and are yellowish greens in color. Hemp seeds have a nutty flavor and are sometimes called hemp hearts.

History

Ancient Egypt has medical records that mentioned using Cannabis as a helpful medication during ancient times *(Rodriguez-Leyva & Pierce, 2010)*. Cannabis sativa is one of the oldest cultivated plants as it provides food, fiber, and oils and has medicinal value.

Ancient Asian sailors utilized hemp fibers for their boats' sails. These same fibers can produce high-quality linen. In China, these hemp fibers are used to make their oldest papers which hold valuable historical documents of their culture. Hemp seed oils are eventually utilized as paint or varnish ingredients. As innovations in research occurred, the health benefits of the hemp seed oil and its differentiation from other Cannabis plants were put into place.

Habitat & Cultivation

Countries like Canada, Australia, China, France, Spain, Austria, and Great Britain have prominent hemp seed production *(Rodriguez-Leyva & Pierce, 2010)*. However, until recently, there were issues regarding the cultivation of hemp seed in the United States. Aside from these legality concerns, hemp plants grow annually in temperate regions. They need at least 6 hours of direct sunlight and well-draining soil to thrive.

Active Compounds: Polyunsaturated fatty acid (70–90%) – alpha-linolenic acid, gamma-linolenic acid, linoleic acid; Omega-6 and Omega-3 fatty acids at a three to one (3:1) ratio (50-70%)

Herbal Actions: Anti-inflammatory

Parts Used: Seeds (All parts of the plant are valuable)

Main Use:

- Lowers blood pressure
- Improves heart health
- Hormone balance
- Pain reliever
- Age-related brain function decline
- Digestive health
- Diabetes

Self-care Use:

- Moisturize and condition skin
- PMS and menstrual cramps (gamma-linolenic acid)
- Promotes weight (gamma-linolenic acid may reduce sugar cravings)
- Arthritis (gamma-linolenic acid reduces inflammation)
- Improves brain function (Omega-6 and Omega-3)
- Pregnancy (Omega-3 essential in fetal growth of the brain and retina)

⚠ **Caution!**

★ DO NOT take hemp seed oil if you have low blood pressure or are taking medication for low blood pressure.

★ Check with your doctor if you are PREGNANT or plan to become pregnant. (Blood pressure may lower during pregnancy).

★ Check with your doctor if you are going to have surgery. They may have you stop taking hemp seed oil for a period of time before and after surgery.

Holy Basil

Ocimum tenuiflorum (Lamiaceae)

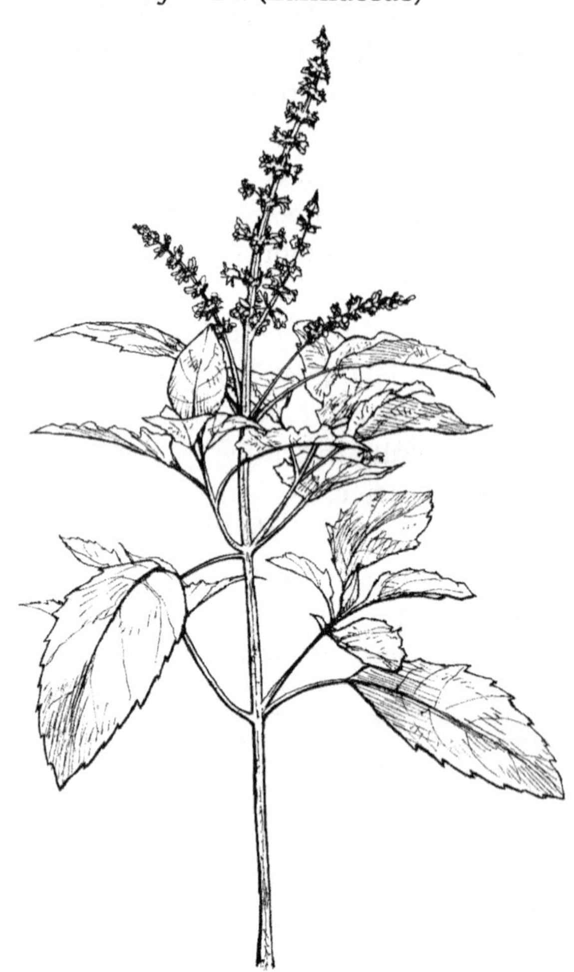

Holy basil (tulsi in Hindi) is a tonic herb that can promote optimal health by revitalizing an individual's mind and body. Every part of this versatile herb is used to target a particular health concern *(Krans, 2020)*. For instance, its leaves and seeds contain active components that help manage malaria. Alcoholic extraction gets compounds that may alleviate stomach issues and eye diseases. For insect bites, essential oils from holy basil may ease the discomfort. Moreover, it may promote health by helping you cope with stress, detoxify the body, and reduce blood sugar.

My friend's grandfather had diabetes and regularly suffered from bouts of hyperglycemia. I told her about holy basil and how it might be a healthy alternative to try. She went to a herbarium I recommended, where she purchased a holy basil tincture. It was only a few weeks before she called to tell me her grandfather was feeling better than he had in years. He now tells anyone who will listen about how holy basil changed his life.

Description

Holy basil is an aromatic annual or short-lived perennial shrub. Their stalks are fuzzy and grow to about 3 feet (1 meter) tall. Depending on the variety, the flowers are dark purple or light green and produce small rust-colored fruit. The leaves are ovate with slightly ridged edges and have soft short hairs on both sides.

History

Ancient practitioners believed that this plant's healing powers helped them manage numerous health issues commonly encountered by ancient civilizations. Indian medicine used this herb for eye diseases and to treat parasitic ringworms *(Krans, 2020)*. Because of the rich uses of holy basil, the Ayurveda medical system even referred to it as the "elixir of life" *(Jamshidi & Cohen, 2017)*. They believed it could balance one's mind, body, and spirit.

Habitat & Cultivation

Native to Southeast Asia and India, holy basil grows well in tropical and subtropical areas. Because of its history, religious Indian communities continue to plant holy basil around places of worship.

Whether you grow holy basil from seed, cutting, or transplanted seedling, it is easy to grow this herb at home. Germinate your seeds indoors 6–8 weeks before the season's last frost. If you live in warmer climates, you can start them outside. You should keep the soil moist but not saturated until the seeds germinate.

Active Compounds: Flavonoids (apigenin, luteolin); Volatile oil (1%) — eugenol (70–80%); Triterpene (unsolicited acid); Polyphenols (rosmarinic acid); Saponins; Vitamins and minerals (vitamin C, iron, calcium, and zinc)

Herbal Actions: Adaptogen; Analgesic; Anti-inflammatory; Antispasmodic; Lowers blood sugar levels; Reduces fever

Parts Used: Aerial parts (dried or fresh)

Main Use:

- Diabetes
- Strengthening the immune system
- Anticancer properties
- Protects the heart from stress

Self-care Use:

- Bites and stings
- Respiratory: asthma; cold, coughs, bronchitis and pleurisy

⚠ **Caution!**

★ DO NOT use holy basil if you are PREGNANT or plan to become pregnant.
★ MAY inhibit sperm production

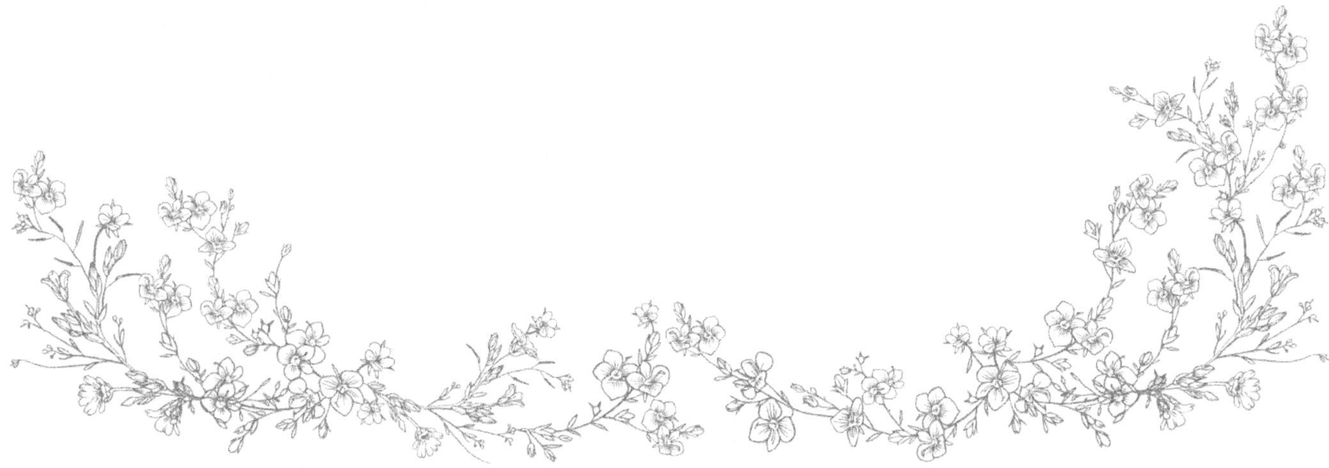

Hops

Humulus lupulus (Cannabaceae)

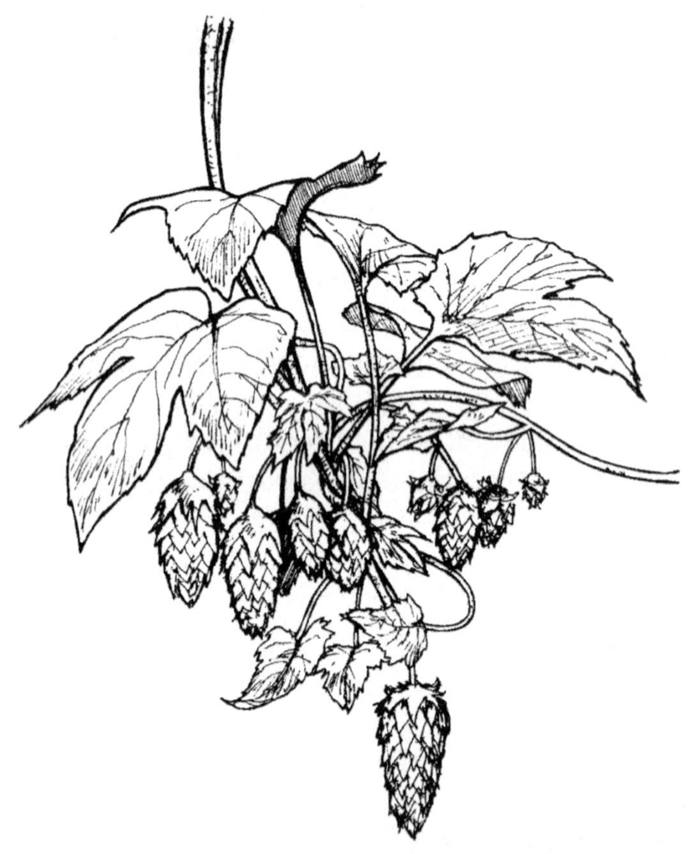

Hops are most commonly known for being the plant that beer comes from, but researchers have also been looking deeper into the possible medicinal benefits of this herb. One of the most known effects of hops is its ability to promote sleep and help manage insomnia *(Butler, 2019)*. The effects of this plant are boosted if mixed with similar sedative-like herbs such as valerian.

One day, a coworker was chatting with me about their child's recent attention deficit hyperactivity disorder (ADHA) diagnosis. She knew I dabbled with herbalism and asked if I knew any safe herbs for kids. I suggested she look into hops extract. She was apprehensive, at first, until she went home and did the research herself. Now her child has been taking hops extract regularly for years. Every time I see her, she thanks me for introducing her to this fantastic herb.

Description

The hops plant is described as climbing vines with stiff hairs that allow it to grow downward. The vines can grow up to 25 feet (7.62 meters) long and have flowers with a yellow-green color. Like the cannabis herb, there are both male and female hops plants (dioecious). The male plant has loose flower bunches, while the female has flowers resembling tiny pinecones. Hidden inside each ripe female flower are yellow pod-like glands called lupulin, the crucial component used in herbal formulas.

History

Historical uses of hops include mainly European herbal practices. King George III (1738–1820) was said to use bedding filled with hops to help him sleep. Historical studies in France (1813) isolated the active compound of lupulin and praised its sleep-inducing virtues *(Koetter & Biendl, n.d.)*. Hops were also traditionally used by many Native Americans for ailments ranging from coughs and colds to gastric disturbances.

Habitat & Cultivation

Hops are perennial flowering plants that bloom after they reach their optimal height. Although male plants are needed for breeding, female flowers are essential when cultivating. They are harvested before ripening and dried. *(Koetter & Biendl, n.d.)*. Hops need a location that can accommodate their growth pattern. They like deep, sandy loam soil that is well draining.

Active Compounds: Bitter (lupulin humulon, lupulon and valerianic acid); Flavonoids; Estrogenic tannins; Polyphenolic tannins; Volatile oil (1%), humulene

Herbal Actions: Antispasmodic; Aromatic bitters; Sedative; Soporific

Parts Used: Strobilus cone (dried or fresh)

Main Use:

- Bitter: Strong stimulant for digestion; Sedative (lupulin); Antiseptic (lupulon and humulon)
- Sedative: Calms the mind; Reduces restlessness and irritability; Helps promote sound sleep
- Antispasmodic: Stress, anxiety, and tension headaches; Certain types of asthma; Menstrual pains

Self-care Use:

- Insomnia: Relaxes smooth muscle
- Aids digestion

⚠ **Caution!**

★ DO NOT take if you have depression or are prone to depressive states

★ DO NOT use hops if you have hormone-sensitive conditions or cancers. Hop contains chemical compounds that mimic estrogen.

★ Women may see changes in menstruation cycles

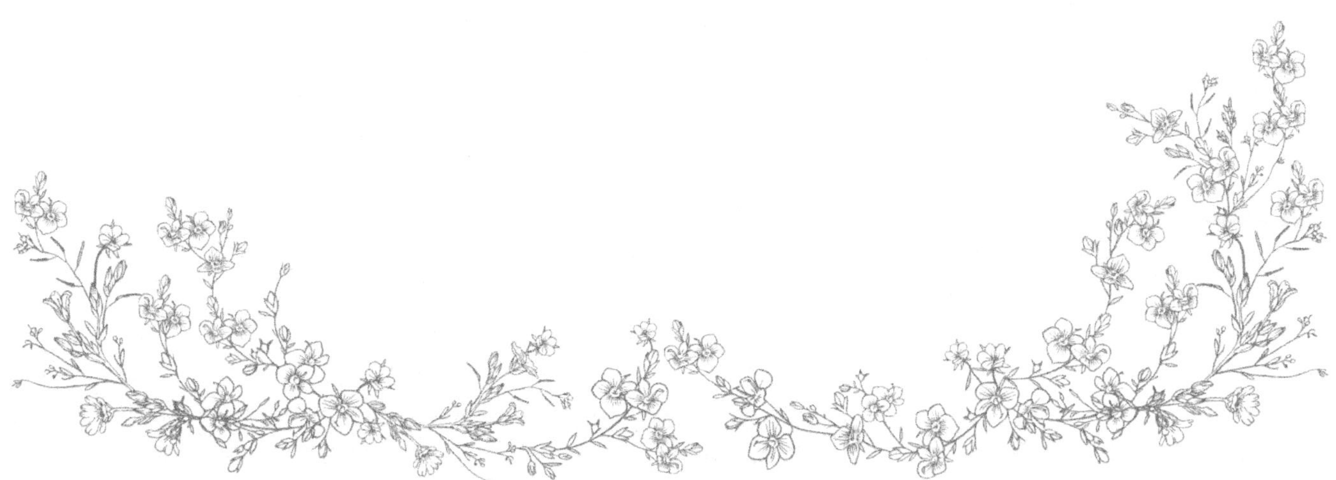

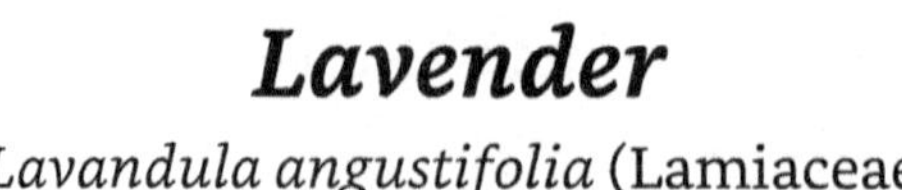

Lavender

Lavandula angustifolia (Lamiaceae)

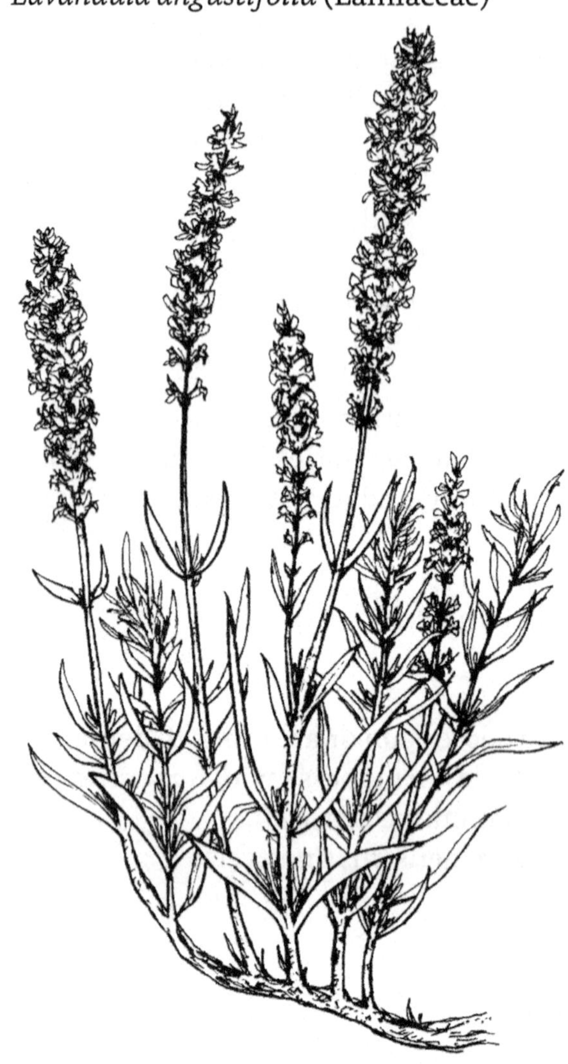

Lavender is primarily cultivated to extract essential oils by distilling its flower spikes. Lavender oil is a key ingredient in many cosmetic products for its clarifying properties and fragrance. This distinct fragrance is relaxing and used in aromatherapy to help with insomnia, depression, and stress management *(Nordquist, 2019)*. Aside from these, lavender may also provide anti-inflammatory and antiseptic properties to assist with minor bug bites and simple wound healing.

I can not get enough of this herb! I use it in Epsom salt baths and frequently make infused tea blends with lavender. It also gained popularity in my local coffee shop a few years back, and a friend talked me into getting a lavender latte one day. I was highly impressed. As long as the barista goes easy on the infused syrup, it gives a subtle aromatic sweetness to any hot beverage.

Description

Lavender is a small branching shrub with gray-green leaves and elongated shoots or spikes containing lilac or blue flowers. These spikes are around 8–16 inches (20–40 centimeters) long. The lavender herb can grow to about 1.3 feet (0.4 meters) tall and live for 30 years!

History

Lavender originated from the Mediterranean region, the Middle East, and India. The history of lavender was mainly associated with love. For example, Cleopatra used lavender to seduce Julius Caesar and Mark Antony *(Perry, 2019).* Women during the early civilizations even wore small pouches filled with lavender to lure in suitors.

Aside from those, lavender's historical applications include warding off evil spirits *(Perry, 2019).* We now know that lavender may have antimicrobial properties and that the "evil spirits" might have been certain diseases associated with inflammation, stress, and anxiety.

Habitat & Cultivation

Lavender's primary habitat is Northern Africa and the mountains of the Mediterranean. The flowers are only harvested when they obtain the components needed in the extraction procedure. Usually, this is the season toward the end of the flowering phase.

Growing this herb at home may take a little tender loving care. The seeds take a long time to germinate, and plants may not produce flowers in the first year. They do not reach full maturity for about three years. For this reason, most lavender is propagated by cutting the root from a mature plant. Make sure your plants have plenty of sunlight and well-draining soil.

Active Compounds: Flavonoids; Volatile oil (up to 3%); Linalyl acetate (30–60%); Cineole (10 %); Linalool; Nerol; Borneol

Herbal Actions: Antidepressant; Antispasmodic; Antimicrobial; Neuroprotective

Parts Used: Flowers (dried or fresh)

Main Use:

- Relieves sleeplessness
- Alleviates depression
- Helps with irritability
- Soothes indigestion, gas, bolting, and colic
- Effective for some types of asthma
- Relieves muscle tension

Self-care Use:

- Back pain; Stiff and achy joints; Neuralgia
- Bites, stings, burns, and sunburns
- Earaches
- Headaches and migraines
- Insomnia

⚠ Caution!

★ DO NOT use essential oil internally (only under doctor supervision)

★ Essential oil applied to the skin may cause irritation in some cases.

★ Allergic reactions may happen. Discontinue use if you start feeling nauseous, experience vomiting, or have increased headaches.

Lemon Balm

Melissa officinalis (Lamiaceae)

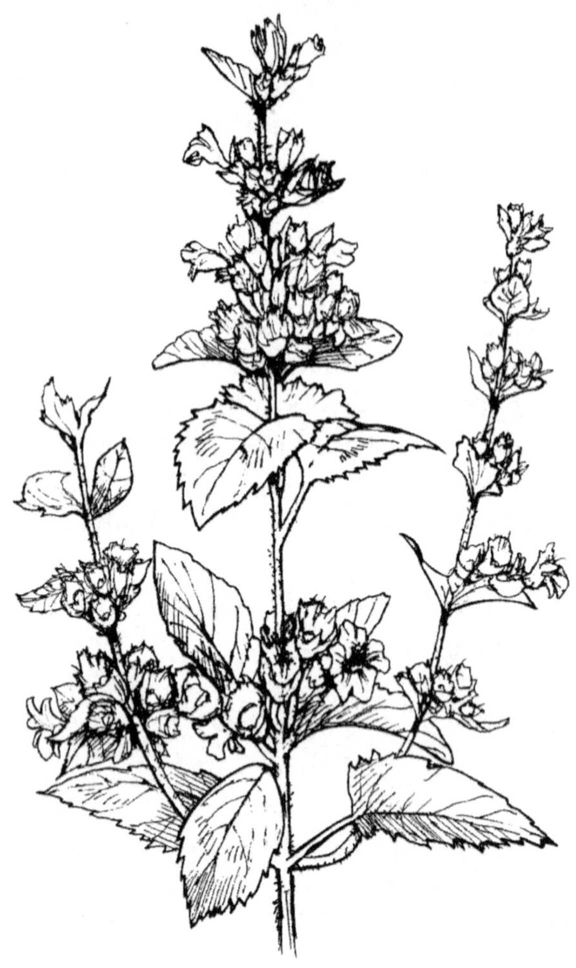

Lemon balm adds aroma and flavor to marinated meat, baked goods, and jam. It is excellent for making syrup infusions to spruce up a glass of iced tea or add to cocktails. You can also just put a few sprigs in your sun tea jar to enjoy its stress-relieving qualities. If you struggle with stress, sleep problems, or anxiety, lemon balm may help you with its relaxing effect and mood-boosting capacity. Also, lemon balm is noted to promote cognitive improvement.

Description

Lemon balm is a bushy perennial herb belonging to the mint family and has a distinct lemony aroma. It can grow to about 2.8 feet (80 centimeters) high with leaves that grow opposite on square-shaped stems. The heart-shaped leaves are bright green on top, while the underneath is a whitish color. The white flowers are so tiny that you might not even be able to see them at first glance.

History

With its strong-scented leaves, lemon balm was initially used to entice bees to feed. In fact, its scientific name "*Melissa*" came from the Latin origin "melissóphyllon" or "bee leaf." During past civilizations, lemon balm has been used to manage nervous problems, insect bites, and common colds *(MBC, n.d.)*. Arab practitioners used this herb to help strengthen the heart and treat depressed moods.

Habitat & Cultivation

Although the plant originated in the Eastern Mediterranean and West Asia, you may see lemon balm growing in any region. The best location for this plant to thrive is in sunny and elevated areas around 1000 meters above sea level.

The cultivation of lemon balm at home is similar to other plants in the mint family. Keeping them in the sunlight for at least five hours daily with well-draining soil will allow them to thrive. Watering them daily in summer heat also keeps the plant nourished. They can be a little invasive if not well pruned, but planting them in pots or containers will alleviate this problem.

Active Compounds: Flavonoids; Polyphenols; Tannins; Triterpenes; Volatile oil (up to 2%) citrate, caryophyllene oxide, linalool and citronellal

Herbal Actions: Antispasmodic; Antiviral; Carminative; Increase sweating; Nerve tonic; Relaxant

Parts Used: Aerial parts (dried or fresh)

Main Use:

- Polyphenols: may heal sores from herpes simplex virus in about five days and reduce outbreaks.
- Volatile oil: Strong antispasmodic; Citral and citronellal calm the central nervous system
- Inhibits thyroid function (used for overactive thyroid)
- Relieves heart palpitations and quiet a racing heart

Self-care Use:

- Anxiety, mild depression, and restlessness
- Cold sores, shingles, and chickenpox
- Flu with muscle aches, pains, and fever
- Stomachaches; Nausea caused by emotional problems
- Toothaches

⚠ **Caution!**

- ★ DO NOT use essential oil internally (only under doctor supervision)
- ★ DO NOT take lemon balm if you are taking sedatives or thyroid medications. Talk to your doctor before taking it.

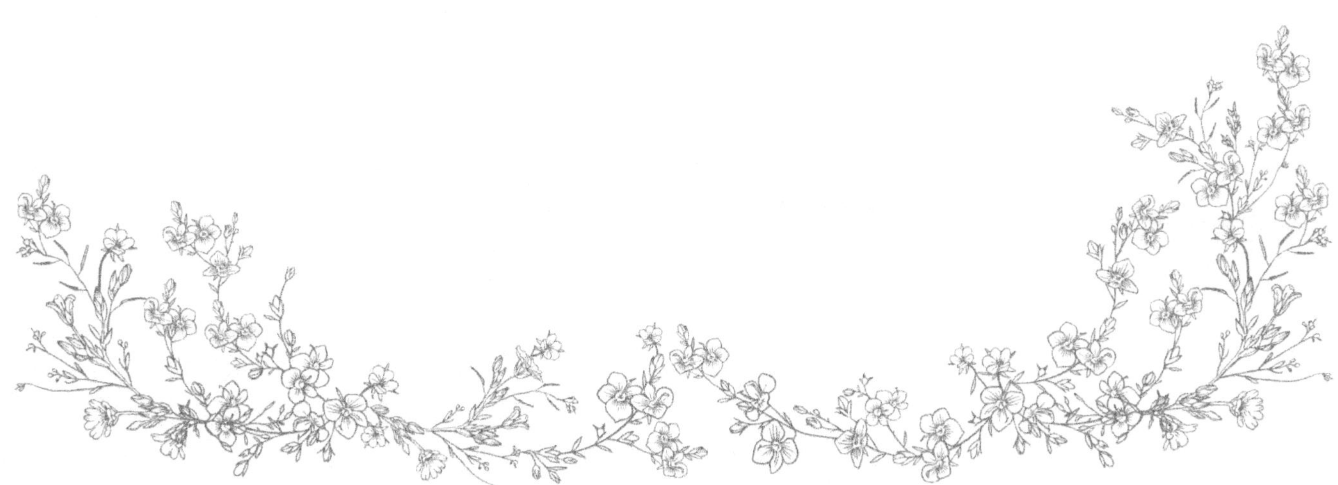

Oregano

Origanum vulgare (Lamiaceae)

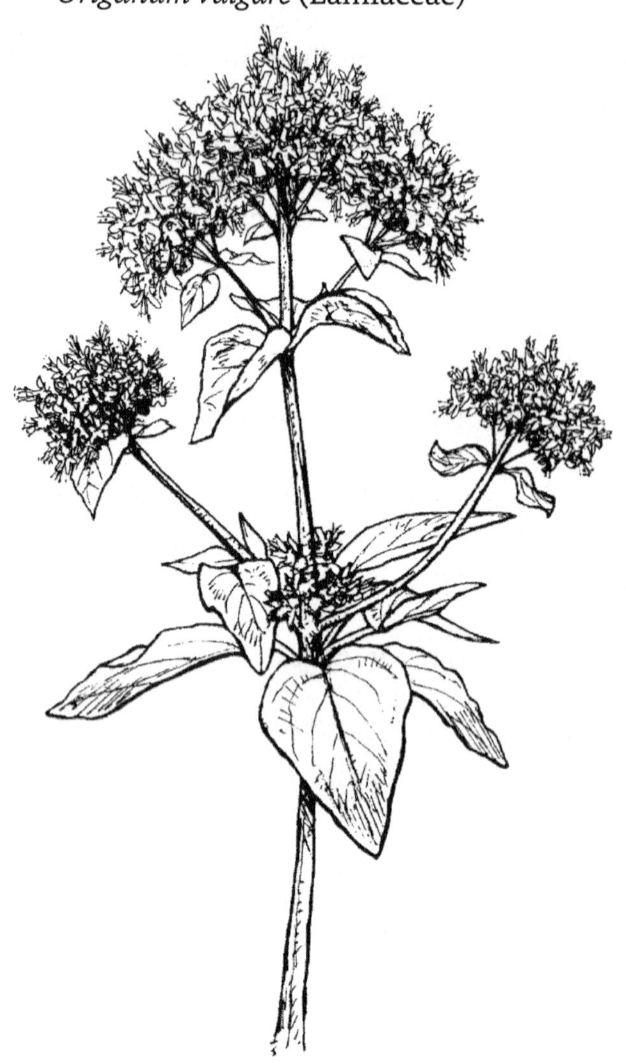

Aside from its dried leaves, essential oils from oregano pack a lot of antioxidants. This herb also has antimicrobial and antifungal properties, which may help you lose weight, lessen your harmful cholesterol levels, and optimize your gut health *(Rowles, 2020)*. Due to its fantastic health benefits, you can buy oregano oil in capsule or tablet forms.

I recommend oregano remedies during cold and flu season to help the immune system. Taken regularly, it can stave off any chances of infection when everyone around you is sick. I take 600 milligrams of oregano oil in capsule form, but you can also brew a soothing herbal infusion blend of oregano, cinnamon, and clove for all your antioxidant needs.

Description

Oregano is a bushy, woody-branched perennial, and just like all members of the mint family, it is characterized by its square stem. These stems can be slightly hairy when the plant is young but become woody when it ages. This herb can grow up to 3 feet (1 meter) tall and around 2 feet (slightly over a half meter) wide. Some varieties of its leaves are fuzzy, but most are coarse, aromatic, and round to ovate-shaped. Once the plant goes to seed, it will be adorned with white or rose-purple flowers.

History

Oregano was well-used by the Greeks and Roman empires to manage skin sores, relieve muscle aches, and provide an organic antiseptic *(Singletary, 2010)*. In Ancient Greece, oregano was infused in remedies to aid optimal health for upset stomachs and common colds. Because of the usefulness and effectiveness of this herb, it was named after the Greek words "oros" (mountain) and "ganos" (joy).

Habitat & Cultivation

Originally, oregano was cultivated in Mediterranean regions, but it is now grown worldwide. Mild climates cater to the growing needs of an oregano plant. You can quickly produce your own from seeds or cuttings, but make sure to plant them where they can get a generous amount of sunlight.

Active Compounds: Volatile oil (carvacrol, beta-bisabolene, caryophyllene, thymol, borneol, and linalool); Flavonoids; Resin; Sterols; Tannins

Herbal Actions: Antibacterial; Antifungal; Antioxidant

Parts Used: Aerial parts, essential oil

Main Use:

- Potent antiseptic for bacteria and fungus (Candida and E. coli)
- Infections of the respiratory and gastrointestinal tracts

Self-care Use:

- Diluted essential oil for toothaches and achy joints
- Bronchitis, coughs, and tonsillitis
- Gastroenteritis and dysentery

⚠ **Caution!**

★ DO NOT use essential oil internally (only under doctor supervision)
★ External application may irritate the skin.
★ DO NOT take if you have a vitamin K deficiency or suffer from blood clotting
★ DO NOT take as a medicine during PREGNANCY

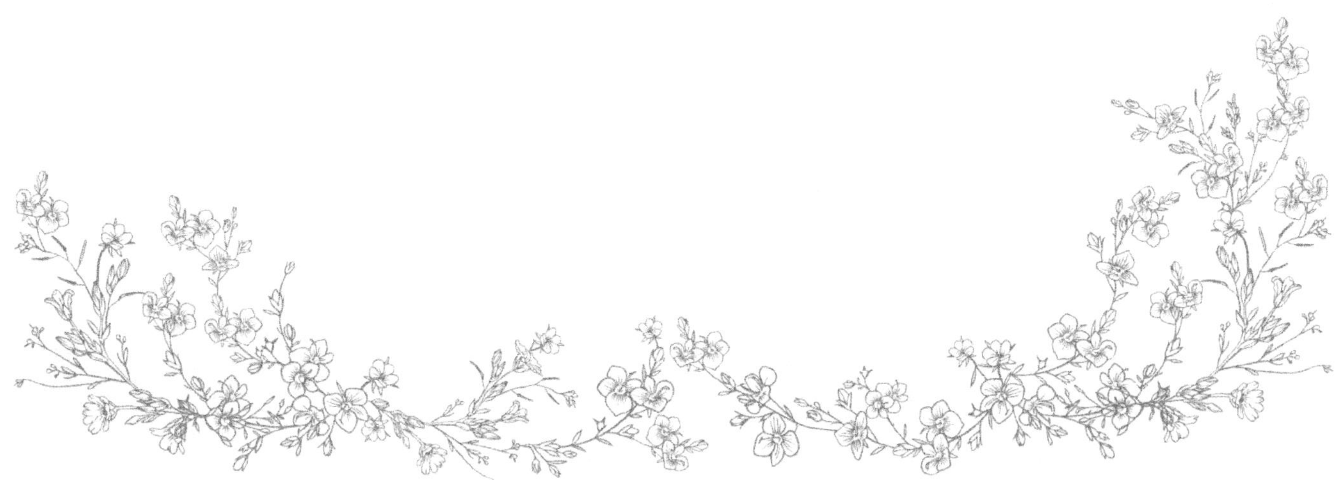

Parsley

Petroselinum crispum (Apiaceae)

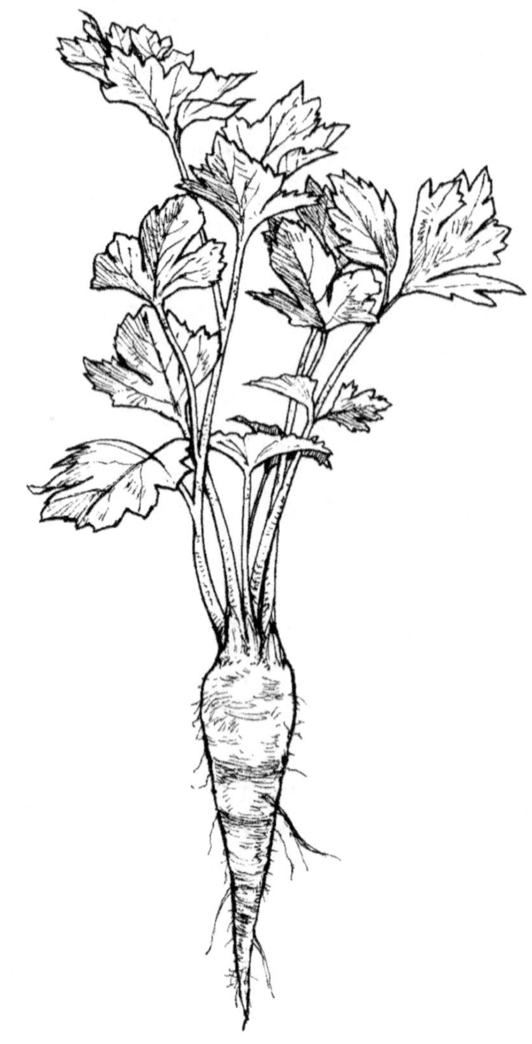

Parsley is particularly rich in vitamin K – a vitamin that supports healthy bones and blood clotting *(Zamarripa, 2019)*. It is also rich in antioxidants and flavonoids that may help reduce your risk of developing cancer, diabetes, and heart-related ailments. It is also a fantastic astringent and can aid with detoxing your body.

I have a long history with parsley that goes back to when I had kidney stones. Its astringent quality aided in breaking down the stone and allowed me to pass it. If you need help detoxing or passing stones, I strongly suggest brewing a parsley infusion. Add a teaspoon of dandelion root powder to increase the power of this remedy. It is also suitable for chronic bladder infections!

Description

Parsley can grow to about 34.5 inches (80 centimeters) tall, with stems that are hollow and flavorful enough to eat. The leaves are dark green, flat, or curled, with slightly pointed edges resembling small maple leaves. Whether fresh or dried, it provides a mild peppery flavor that compliments most cuisines.

History

The Hebrews saw parsley as sacred, and the herb was used to celebrate Passover. To this day, they hold this herb in high regard. Parsley was also considered sacred by the Ancient Greeks. According to Greek legends, as the hero Archemorus was eaten by serpents, parsley sprang out from the blood he had shed *(RDF, 2015)*. The sacredness of parsley for the Ancient Greeks prompted them never to place the herb on their tables. Instead, they used parsley as decoration for tombs and as wreaths to crown winners of the Olympians.

Habitat & Cultivation

Parsley is a flowering herb mainly native to Mediterranean regions, but growing this herb in your home garden can be an easy task. It grows well at about 44.6–60.8 °F (7–16 °C), in bright sunlight or under partial shade. All you need to do is sow its seeds in well-draining loamy soil and provide general care and maintenance.

Active Compounds: Flavonoids; Phthalides; Coumarins; Volatile oil (about 20% myristicin, about 18% apiole, and many other terpenes)

Herbal Actions: Anti-inflammatory; Antioxidant; Astringent; Diuretic (volatile oil — specifically myristicin and apiole); Strong uterine stimulant; Menstrual stimulant

Parts Used: Leaves, seeds, and roots

Main Use:

- Seeds used for gout (removes waste from inflamed joints and the kidneys)
- Root used for cystitis, flatulence, and rheumatic conditions

Self-care Use:

- Stimulates delayed menstrual cycle and eases period pain
- Kidney stones (add a ½ teaspoon of dandelion root powder to parsley tea to help dissolve stones)

⚠ **Caution!**

- ★ ☠ DO NOT consume excessive amounts of the seed. TOXIC!
- ★ DO NOT consume the seeds during PREGNANCY or if you have kidney disease.

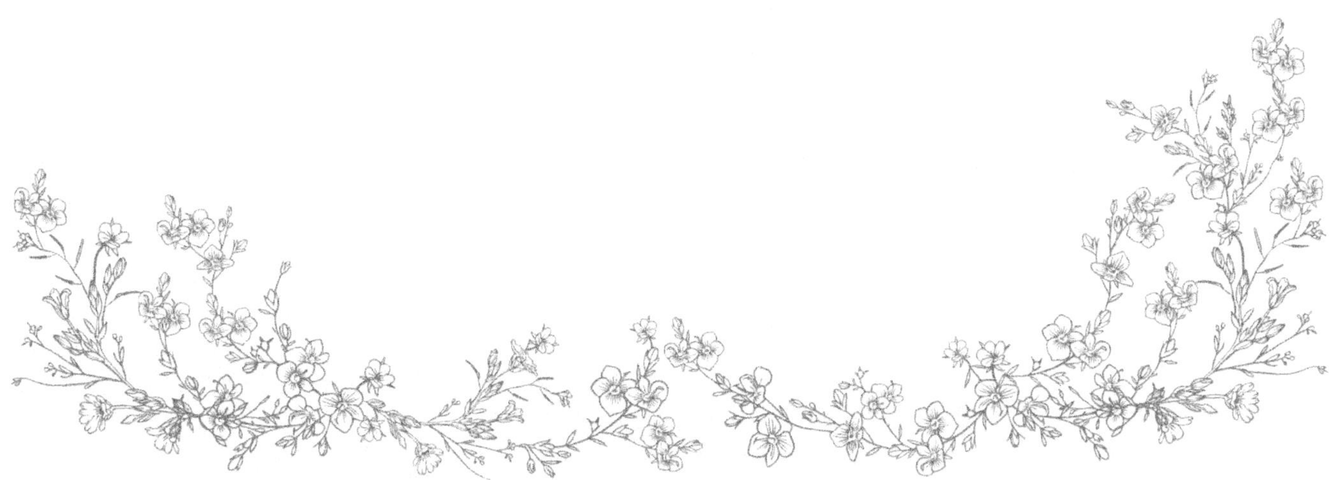

Passionflower

Passiflora caerulea (Passifloraceae)

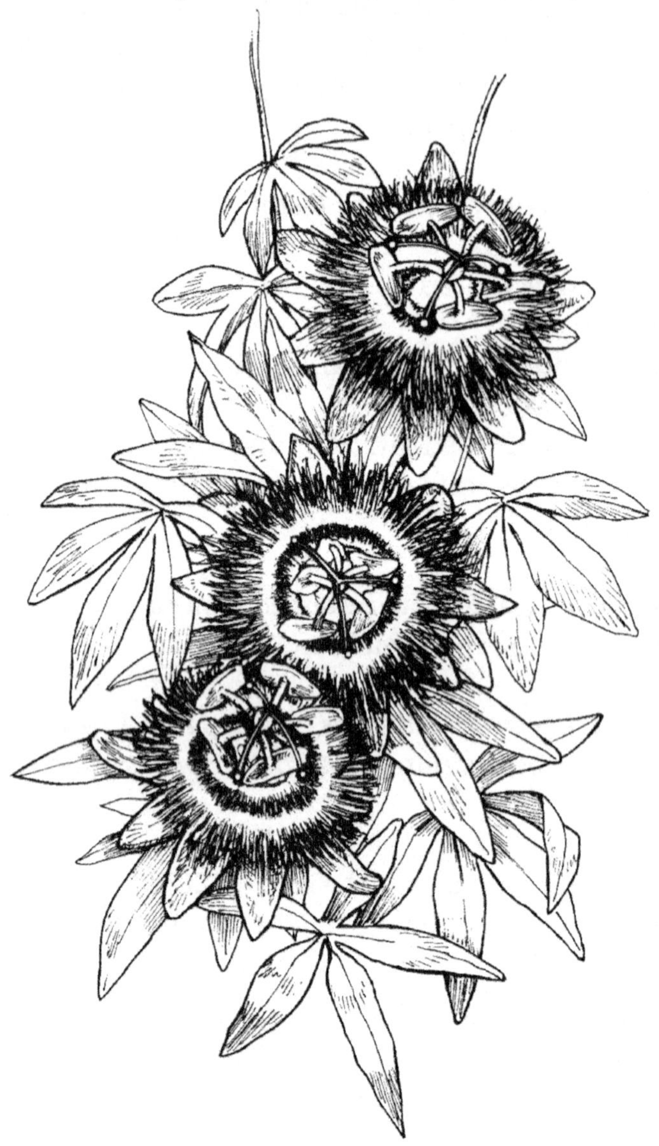

Passionflower has a sedative effect that makes it helpful in managing anxiety and insomnia. It has been known to increase your brain's gamma-aminobutyric acid (GABA) production, which may help suppress pain *(Stinson, 2018)*. GABA is a hormone that helps counteract the excitatory part of your brain, helping you calm down.

To take advantage of the effects of this herb, you can make an herbal infusion by boiling the dried flowers. It is marketed as prepackaged tea, extracts, tablets, or capsules. Do not hesitate to make tablets or capsules yourself. The suggested dosage is about 300–400 milligrams twice a day for no longer than eight weeks.

Description

There are more than 550 different variations of passionflower. The plant is usually a climbing vine with grasping tendrils, but it can also be seen as a tree or shrub, depending on the species. A key identifier is the leaves, which are deeply lobed, finger-like, and grow in groups of three or five. These lobed leaves are either a pointed ovate shape or oblong and grow about 3–8 inches (7.6–20.3 centimeters) long.

The flowers come in various colors, including shades of purple, blue, pink, and yellow. They are probably one of the most unusual-looking flowers found in nature. The blossom's trumpet-shaped tubes have crimped or wavy thread-like filaments that spring from the center tube. The flowers can be petite or large and showy, depending on the variety.

History

During the era of exploration, Spanish sailors were introduced to passionflower by the natives of Peru. The sailors named the plant since they noticed its resemblance to the crucifix. Knowing the Christian background of the Spaniards, they called the plant "passionflower" since "The Passion" pertained to Christ's crucifixion and final hours.

Historically, Native Americans used passionflower to treat liver problems, wounds, and boils *(Ashpari, 2018)*. Meanwhile, Europeans utilized this herb to manage restlessness and anxiety.

Habitat & Cultivation

Most passionflower species are native to the Southeastern United States. This region has sandy soils with low moist woody areas, which passionflowers prefer. You may also find them growing on rocky cliffs, on the side of a road, or crawling up fence lines.

If you want to grow this plant at home, I suggest using a trellis or fence because they tend to die if they remain on the ground. All passionflower variations need plenty of sunlight and well-draining soil. They appreciate partial shade if cultivated in especially hot regions and grow relatively fast.

Active Compounds: Amino acids; Cyanogenic glycosides (gynocardin); Flavonoids (apigenin); Indole alkaloids (trace)

Herbal Actions: Antispasmodic; Genial sedative; Tranquilizing

Parts Used: Aerial parts (dried or fresh)

Main Use:

- Short term sleeplessness and insomnia
- Anxiety, irritability, and tension
- Non-addictive herbal tranquilizer
- Pain reliever

Self-care Use:

- Insomnia
- Sleeplessness due to backaches
- Toothaches, headaches, and menstrual pains

⚠ **Caution!**

- ★ DO NOT take high doses during PREGNANCY
- ★ DO NOT take it in conjunction with other sedatives. Doing so may cause excessive drowsiness.

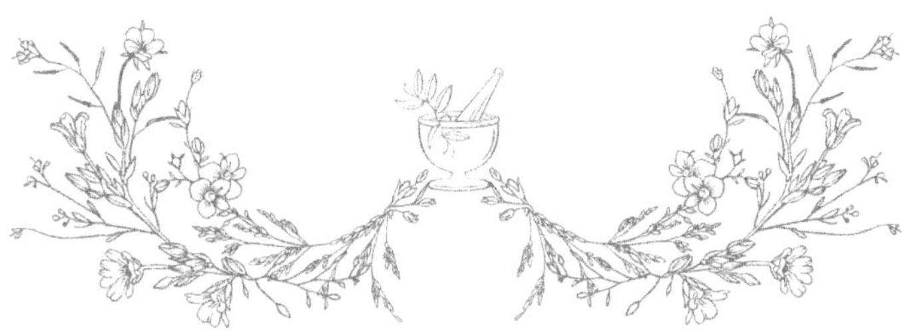

Rosemary

Rosmarinus officinalis (Lamiaceae)

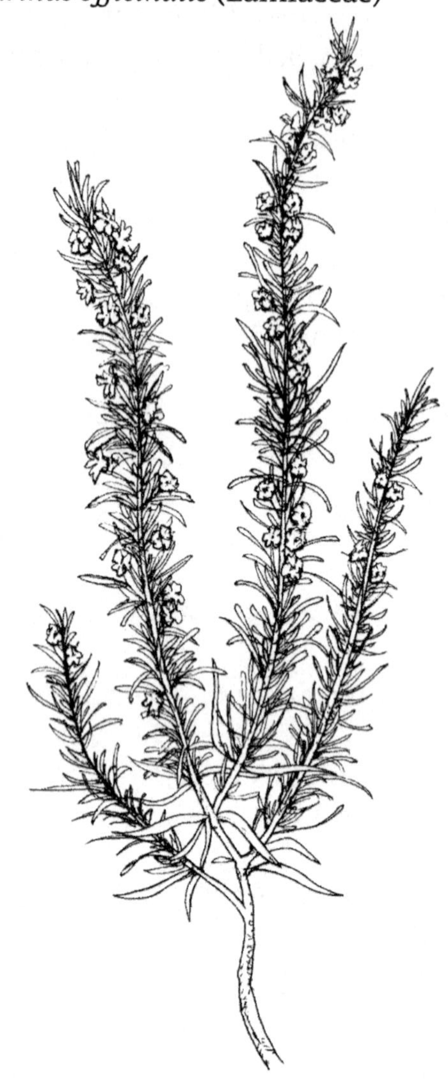

Rosemary is an aromatic shrub with typical culinary applications and herbal benefits. Finely mincing rosemary leaves can make a more flavorful soup, stew, or pasta. It also is used in some food preservation processes. Aside from its culinary uses, rosemary has many medicinal properties.

Essential oils extracted from rosemary leaves are used in folk medicine to aid cognitive function, stimulate hair growth, relieve pain, ease stress, and even repel bugs *(McCulloch, 2018)*. I like to utilize a rosemary tincture to alleviate muscle strain after a long workout and to boost circulation.

Description

Rosemary is a woody, perennial, bushy shrub with needle-like leaves. The leaves are dark green on the top and have short, white, wooly hairs on the underside. The plant can grow to about 6 feet (1.83 meters) tall and 4–5 feet (1.22–1.52 meters) wide. The aroma is a pleasant wooden fragrance, while the taste is peppery, sage-like, with a bitter aftertaste.

History

Ancient herbal practitioners used rosemary as an ingredient in tonics and salves, and it was even believed to help protect individuals from contracting the plague. Also, ancient civilizations saw rosemary as a plant that helped reinforce memory since it slightly stimulates the brain. It was also said to alleviate headaches in most cases.

Habitat & Cultivation

The Mediterranean region is known to be the origin of rosemary. Today it is widely cultivated in numerous parts of Europe, Asia, and Africa. If you want to grow it at home, gardens with warm climates will not have a problem growing this shrub. Ensure you have well-draining sandy soil, and keep your plants in direct sunlight for six to eight hours daily. Rosemary plants do not like cold weather and will wilt in temperatures below 30 °F (-1.11 °C).

Active Compounds: Diterpenes (carnosic acid and carnosol); Flavonoids (apigenin, diosmin); Rosmarinic acid; Tannins; Volatile oil (1–2%) — borneol, camphene, camphor, and cineole

Herbal Actions: Astringent; Anti-inflammatory; Antioxidant; Nervine; Stimulant; Tonic

Parts Used: Leaves (dried or fresh)

Main Use:

- Circulatory stimulant: Increase blood flow, especially for those with low blood pressure; Promoter blood flow to the head, improving memory and concentration
- May help repair nerves
- Aids in recovering from long term stress and chronic illness
- Stimulates adrenal glands

Self-care Use:

- Migraines
- Premenopausal syndrome (PMS)
- Sore throats
- Tired and achy muscles
- Mild to moderate depression

⚠ **Caution!**

★ DO NOT use essential oil internally (only under doctor supervision)

★ Consuming large amounts of rosemary may irritate the stomach and intestines. Doing so could also lead to kidney damage.

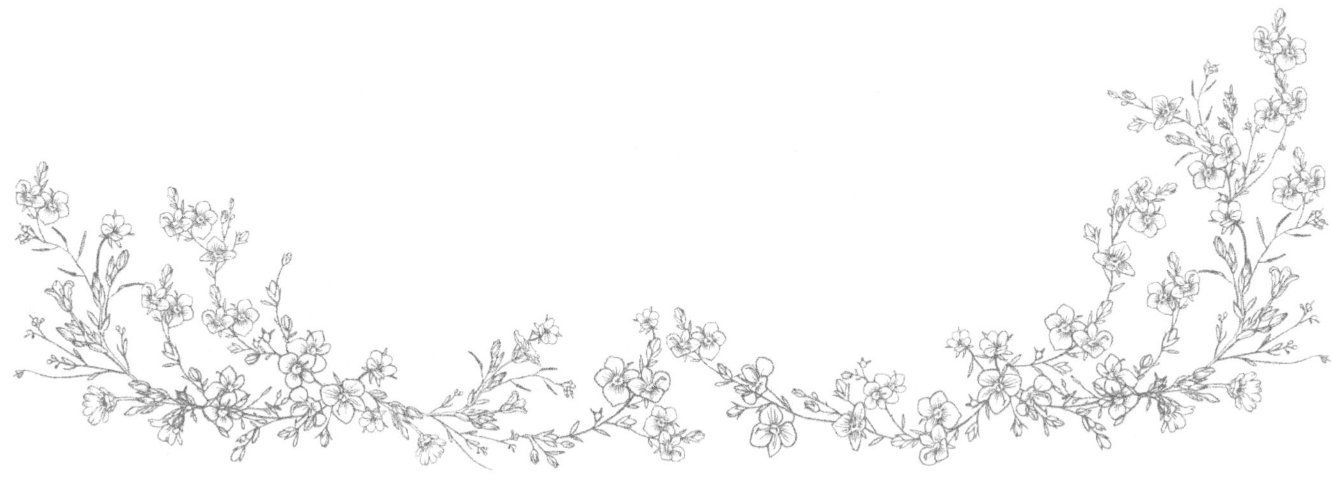

Skullcap

Scutellaria lateriflora (Lamiaceae)

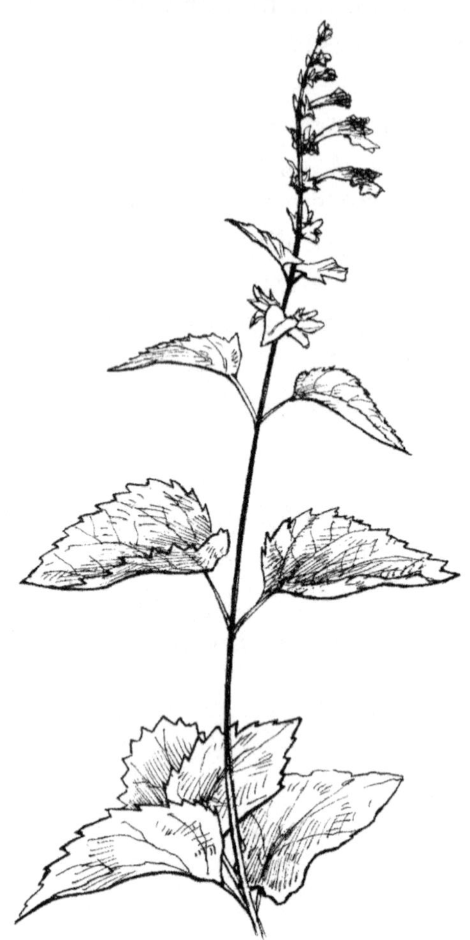

The active components in the skullcap plant are primarily used for sedation or as a sleeping pill ingredient *(Livertox, 2020)*. The aerial parts of skullcap contain massive amounts of flavonoids which can be extracted for their soothing effect. Aside from skullcap extracts, it is also available as powders to make tea and capsules and incorporated in some over-the-counter herbal solutions.

Anxiety and depression can be overwhelming and debilitating; however, there may be a solution for you in the power of skullcap. You will want to read the individual labeling if you purchase a ready-made product, but typically you should not take skullcap remedies longer than two weeks. Try mixing up a skullcap formula at home to chase away those pesky feelings of anxiety and depression.

Description

Skullcap is a perennial that grows between 1–3 feet (31 centimeters to about a meter) tall and is part of the mint family. The leaves are bright green and have jagged edges. This plant has some dish-shaped sepals seen during its fruiting period. The sepals are modified leaves that encase the flowers. The plant's flowers are usually a distinct blue color but can appear in varying shades. They grow in pairs and sprout from one side of the square stems.

History

The odd name of the plant came from the flowers' resemblance to European soldiers' helmets. For numerous centuries skullcap has been used by Native Americans to help in managing menstrual problems, anxiety, and digestive or kidney ailments *(Livertox, 2020).* Today, herbalists and naturopaths still utilize this herb as a sedative, antispasmodic and nervine tonic.

Habitat & Cultivation

Skullcap is found in moist woodland regions of North America, where it is native *(ABC, n.d.)*. Pretty blue flowers may appear around July to September. During this season, the aerial parts are harvested and prepared for an herbal treatment.

It prefers fertile, well-draining soil if you want to grow this plant at home. Make sure to give your plants partial to full sun. The seedlings will sprout faster if you saturate them with water for about a week. You can also start them indoors 6–8 weeks before the last frost and plant them outside after all risk of frost has passed.

Active Compounds: Bitter iridoids (catalpol); Flavonoids (scutellarin); Tannins; Volatile oil

Herbal Actions: Antispasmodic; Mild bitter; Nervine tonic; Sedative

Parts Used: Aerial parts (dried or fresh)

Main Use:

- Flavonoids: Scutellarin can help with anxiety and stress; Mood elevator
- Nerve tonic: Restore and nourish the nervous system
- Antispasmodic: Helps when stress and worry causes muscle tension; Period pain
- Cherokee Native Americans utilize this herb for: Menstrual stimulation; Breast pain; Encourage the placenta to expel

Self-care Use

- Anxiety, panic attacks, and depression
- Migraines, headaches, and tension
- Insomnia

⚠ **Caution!**

★ DO NOT take skullcap without first checking with your doctor!

★ Taking a high dosage of skullcap tincture may cause mental confusion, stupor, irregular heartbeat, twitching, and seizures.

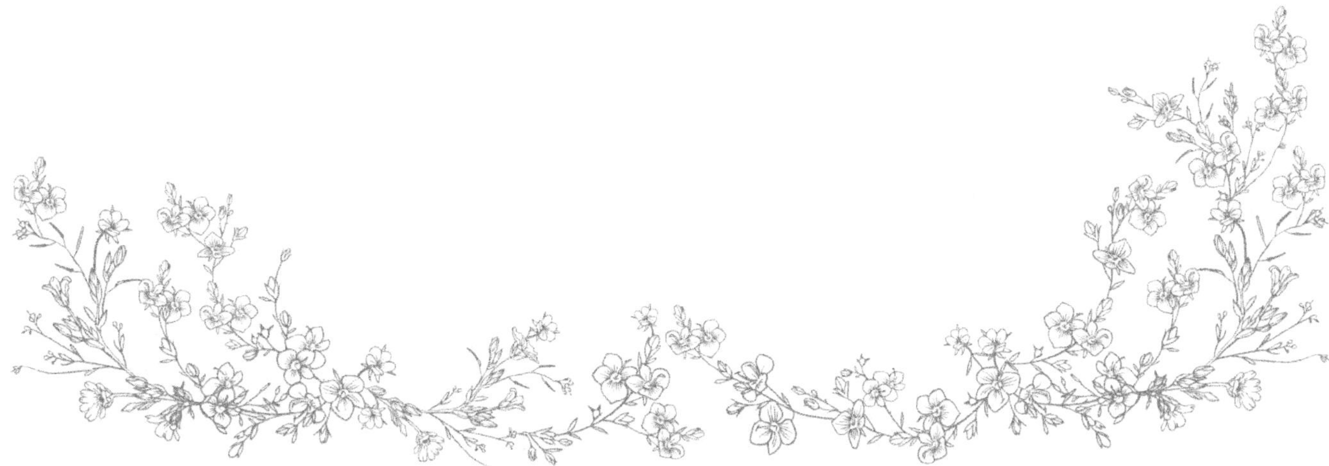

Slippery Elm

Ulmus rubra (Ulmaceae)

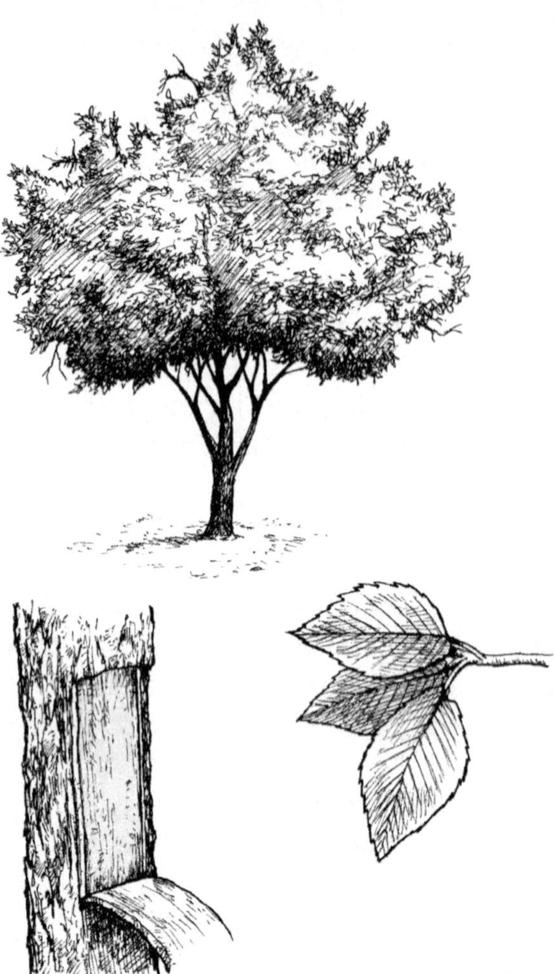

The inner bark of the slippery elm tree is obtained and prepared to help soothe a cough, sore throat, heartburn, and GERD *(Cafasso, 2019)*. The demulcent ability of this bark also helps calm the lining of your digestive tract. You may see slippery elms sold as lozenges, tablets, and powders for making tea or poultice.

I have used this wonderful herb to aid ailments such as burns, boils, abscesses, toothaches, and cold sores. I once gave a slippery elm salve to a friend who had trouble with regular cold sores. It is now the only thing they use when breakouts happen.

Description

Slippery elm is a tree of medium size and can reach up to 80 feet (about 24.4 meters) tall. Wide spreading branches form its crown, filled with long green leaves. The most significant part of the plant is its inner bark. Its gummy and slippery texture is utilized for its added benefits to your holistic wellness.

History

Named for its slippery and mucilaginous inner bark, early North American pioneers used it to help quench their thirst. Eventually, the gummy substance was collected and used for wounds, sore throats, fevers, and many other ailments *(Cafasso, 2019)*. Native American tribes had a wide use for the plant, and later American soldiers utilized slippery elm during the revolution to help their troops suffering from gunshot wounds.

Habitat & Cultivation

Native to North America, this tree loves to have access to full sunlight. Although slippery elm prefers moist and fertile soil near freshwater streams, it can also adapt and tolerate dry soil. These trees also thrive in urban conditions. If you intend to grow them at home, you should ensure they have plenty of space to flourish. Planting them close to structures, like your house, is not advised. The roots may damage sidewalks and building foundations.

Active Compounds: Mucilage; Starch; Tannins

Herbal Actions: Demulcent; Emollient; Nutritive; Laxative

Parts Used: Inner bark (dried or fresh)

Main Use:

- Mucilage: Used to soothe and protect inflamed surfaces both inside and outside the body; Draws out toxins and irritants
- Nutritive: Acts as a probiotic and aids in good gut health
- Acidity, diarrhea, and gastroenteritis
- Inflammation of the gut, constipation, irritable bowel syndrome, colic, diverticulitis, and hemorrhoids
- Urinary issues (chronic cystitis)
- Respiratory system (coughs, chest congestion, tuberculosis, and pleurisy)

Self-care Use

- Acidity and indigestion
- Acne and boils
- Constipation (Children)
- Hemorrhoids

⚠ Caution!

- ★ DO NOT take slippery elm if you are PREGNANT, plan to become pregnant, or breastfeeding.
- ★ May interfere with absorption of other drugs. Take slippery elm at least 2 hours before or after taking medications.

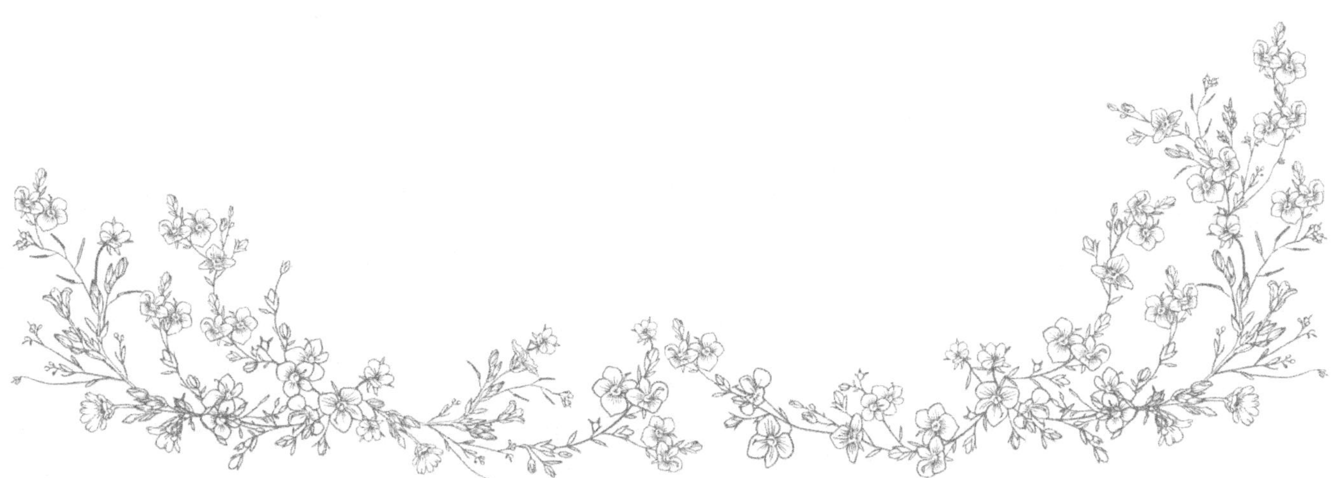

Thyme

Thymus vulgaris (Lamiaceae)

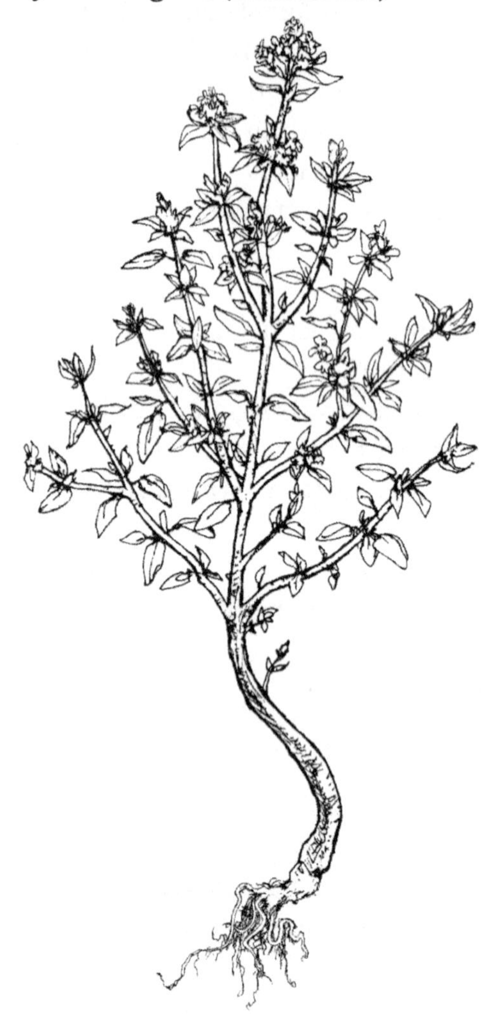

Thyme is an herb you will surely see on shelves alongside other herbs and spices for kitchen use. This herb is a go-to culinary addition to help bring flavor and aroma to your dishes. However, thyme also has medicinal and ornamental uses.

Thymes' antibacterial property makes it very helpful if you struggle with managing acne *(Fanous, 2018)*. It is also filled with vitamins C and A, which may help boost immunity. I remember the first homemade cough syrup I ever made was with thyme. It is a natural expectorant and can help break up congestion so you can get all the mucus out of your lungs.

Description

Thyme plants can grow to around 6–12 inches (15.24–30.48 centimeters). It is a fragrant, low-growing perennial shrub with stiff, woody stems and small, ovate leaves. These leaves are greenish-gray and grow to about ¼ inch (0.635 centimeters) long. The flowers of the thyme shrub have a white or lilac color.

History

Thyme has a rich history that dates back to over 3000 years ago when the ancient Sumerians wrote about its use on clay tablets. They found it helpful as an antiseptic and combined it with pears, figs, and water to create poultices that aided in the healing of wounds.

The Ancient Egyptians used thyme for embalming their loved ones *(Fanous, 2018)*. Furthermore, during the Black Death's peak, people used thyme for embalming the dead and managing the spread of the deadly disease. In contrast, Greeks used thyme as a pleasant scent in their baths, while the Romans dusted their floors with it to deter venomous creatures from entering their homes.

Habitat & Cultivation

Thyme is another spice native to the Mediterranean region, but you can definitely grow this herb at home. Thyme shrubs can be cultivated in a sunny location and need well-draining soil. You can grow it by propagating its seeds, cuttings, or root sections. Just remember that thyme plants love the heat!

Active Compounds: Flavonoids; Phenolic acids; Volatile oil (mostly carvacrol and thymol)

Herbal Actions: Antiseptic; Antifungal; Antioxidant; Expectorant; Expels worms; Relieves muscle spasms

Parts Used: Aerial parts (dried or fresh)

Main Use:

- Volatile oil: Thymol is an effective antifungal, expectorant, and aids in expelling worms.
- Anti-aging: Strong antioxidant that may help protect and preserve higher levels of essential fatty acids in the brain
- Infections: External: bites, stings, sciatica, rheumatic pains, athlete's foot, ringworm, thrush, lice, and scabies; Internal: throat and chest
- Stomach ulcers (antibacterial)
- Menstrual pains
- Asthma and hay fever
- Diluted oil massaged into the scalp encourages hair growth and reverse hair loss.

Self-care Use:

- Allergic rhinitis; Fungal infections
- Back pain; Tired and achy muscles
- Bites and stings
- Cold and flu; Coughs and bronchitis
- Earaches
- Maintaining vitality
- Mild asthma

⚠ **Caution!**

★ DO NOT use essential oil externally during PREGNANCY.

★ Thyme essential oil should NEVER be taken internally.

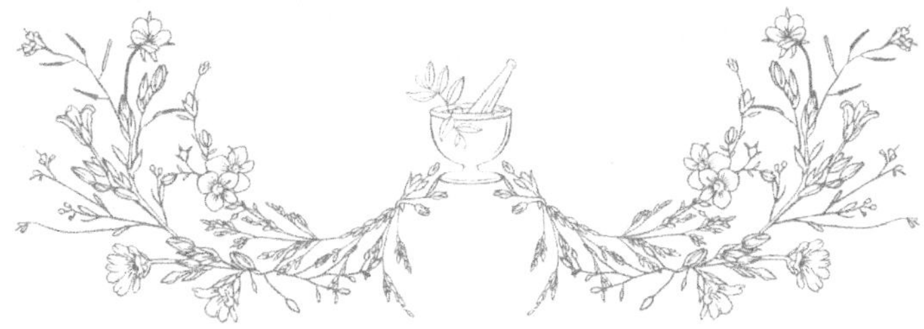

Turmeric

Curcuma longa (Zingiberaceae)

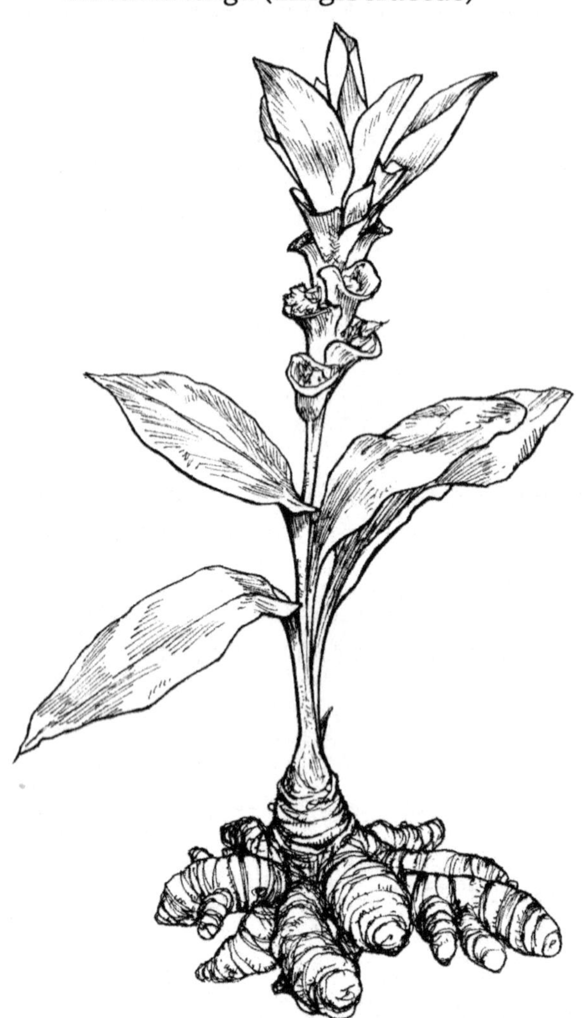

Aside from adding flavor and color to your favorite cuisines, turmeric also has nutritional value and can help the body in multiple ways. Turmeric's most active component is curcumin *(Warwick, 2021)*. This compound can promote wellness in both the body and brain. It reduces the harmful effects of chronic inflammation, lessening your risk of cancer, heart disease, and neurodegenerative problems like Alzheimer's.

Have you ever heard of golden milk? This delicious beverage is one of my favorites to make before bed, especially if I have trouble calming my mind and body. Simmer two cups of milk or milk alternative, about two teaspoons of ground turmeric, and a pinch of black pepper. Adding a little coconut oil or butter to the mix will allow more curcumin to be absorbed into the bloodstream.

Description

Turmeric is a plant in the ginger family, and like ginger, it has herbaceous knobby rhizomes. The plant's rhizomes mature underground as the plant becomes suitable for harvest. Above ground, this perennial plant grows to about 3 feet (around a meter) tall. The leaves are arranged in two rows that alternate along a reed-like stem. The flowers are funnel-like and can be yellow, white, or pink. They bloom between modified leaves in conical-shaped bundles that can grow almost 5 inches (12 centimeters) long.

History

Turmeric was used as early as 4000 years ago by the Indian Vedic culture. This herb had culinary applications and sacred associations. Sanskrit medical treatises and some Ayurvedic records showed turmeric's herbal application in South Asia. The ointment from processing turmeric was used to manage food poisoning *(Benzie & Wachtel-Galor, 2011)*. Furthermore, turmeric was also used by China, East Africa, and Jamaica. The famous explorer, Marco Polo, noted that turmeric was a marvelous discovery similar to saffron.

Habitat & Cultivation

Turmeric herbs are native to tropical climates in south India and Indonesia. The plant prefers to live in temperatures around 68–86 °F (20–30 °C) with a generous amount of rainfall *(Benzie & Wachtel-Galor, 2011)*. The cultivation of this plant is mainly from India. Interestingly, the curcumin component of turmeric from India holds the best quality and highest content compared to those grown in other regions.

Active Compounds: Bitter principles; Curcumin; Resin; Volatile oil (3–5%) — turmerone and zingiberene

Herbal Actions: Anti-inflammatory; Antimicrobial; Anti-platelet (blood-thinning)

Parts Used: Rhizome (dried or fresh)

Main Use:

- Anti-inflammatory: Blocks inflammatory pathways in the body; Arthritis, asthma, psoriasis, and eczema; Taking turmeric with black pepper makes its anti-inflammatory properties more effective.
- Curcumin: Antibacterial (applied to skin and expose to sunlight); Stronger antioxidant than vitamin E
- Supplements may prevent or aid in the treatment of cancers, dementia, and autoimmune diseases.
- Lower cholesterol levels
- Anticoagulant (keeping the blood thin)
- Increases bile production and protects the stomach and liver
- Alleviates nausea, gastritis, and acidity
- Reduces the risk of stroke and heart attacks

Self-care Use:

- Athlete's foot
- Psoriasis
- Nausea and motion sickness

⚠ **Caution!**

★ Turmeric may cause skin irritation

★ DO NOT take if you are taking blood-thinning medications

★ DO NOT take if you have gallstones

Valerian

Valeriana officinalis (Valerianaceae)

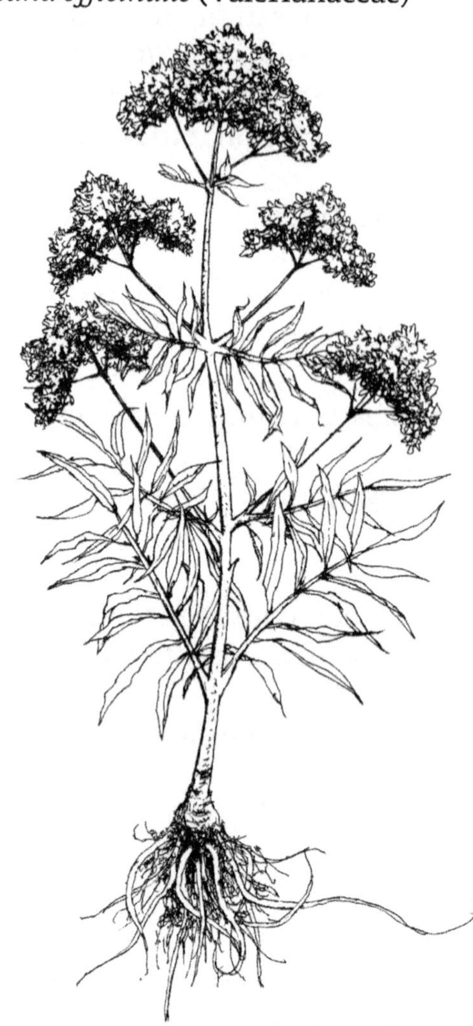

Valerian root is predominantly known for relieving stress and anxiety and improving sleep quality. Fortunately, this herb is safe and well-tolerated, even for children over three. Other benefits include lessening symptoms of PMS and menopause. I use it to alleviate my premenstrual bloating and help calm my emotional state before, during, and after my menstrual cycle.

Description

Valerian is a perennial plant that grows to about 3 feet (1 meter) tall. The stem is straight and hollow with odd-pinnate leaves and lance-shaped leaflets. These leaves are pointed at the tip and slightly hairy underneath. The flowers range from white to pale pink, and the root emits a robust earthy smell. When you bruise the leaves, they release an aromatic scent.

History

The application of valerian root for medicinal use dates back over 2000 years. The scent from its flowers was used as a perfume, while the root was used for traditional medicine. Hippocrates wrote about the therapeutic benefit of this herb, and in the 2nd century, Galen wrote about his prescription of valerian for insomnia.

The name of the plant also has an exciting story. "Valerian" originated from the Latin word "valere," which refers to the phrase "to be strong." This reference may be because this herb is consumed to boost an individual's vitality.

Habitat & Cultivation

Valerian is an herb native to Asia and Europe, but it is currently grown and cultivated in other countries, like the United States and China. The plant can grow in many soil types but typically in a damp, well-drained loam. For the best result at home, plant yours in the sun or partial shade.

Active Compounds: Alkaloids; Iridoids (valepotriates) — valtrate and isovaltrate; Volatile oil (up to 1.4%) — bornyl acetate and beta-caryophyllene

Herbal Actions: Lowers blood pressure; Sedative; Relaxant; Relieves anxiety; Relieves muscle spasms

Parts Used: Root and Rhizome

Main Use:

- Relaxant: Over-contracted muscles (neck and shoulder tension; muscle spasms); Asthma; Colic and irritable bowel syndrome; Period pain
- Anxiety: Tremors, panic, palpitations, and sweating
- Improves sleep (insomnia)
- Stress-related conditions (calming rather than sedative effect)
- High blood pressure

Self-care Use

- Chronic anxiety
- Insomnia
- Nervous exhaustion
- Premenstrual syndrome (PMS)
- Sleeplessness due to backaches

⚠ **Caution!**

★ DO NOT take valerian if you are already taking other sleep-inducing drugs. Can cause excessive drowsiness.
★ May NOT be safe if you are PREGNANT or breast-feeding
★ May NOT be safe for children under the age of three years old

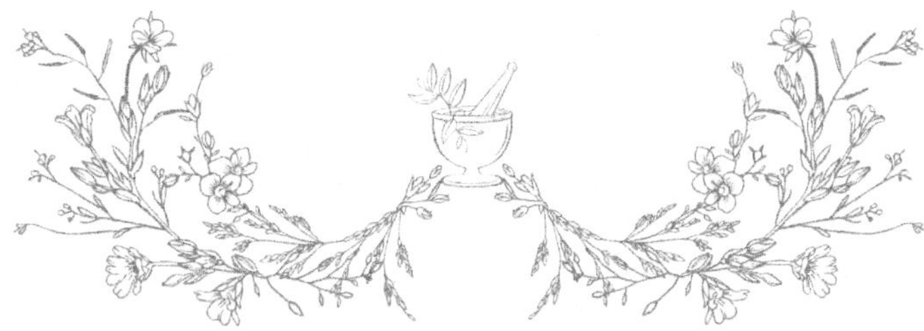

Understanding how herbs can benefit you is the first step in achieving an all-natural journey toward optimal vitality! As you have seen, the benefits of herbs can truly be life-changing as long as you know how to utilize them correctly. Let's take a look at a few more herbs you may want to keep on hand.

Have questions or need support on your herbal journey?

Come Join Our Herbal Family!

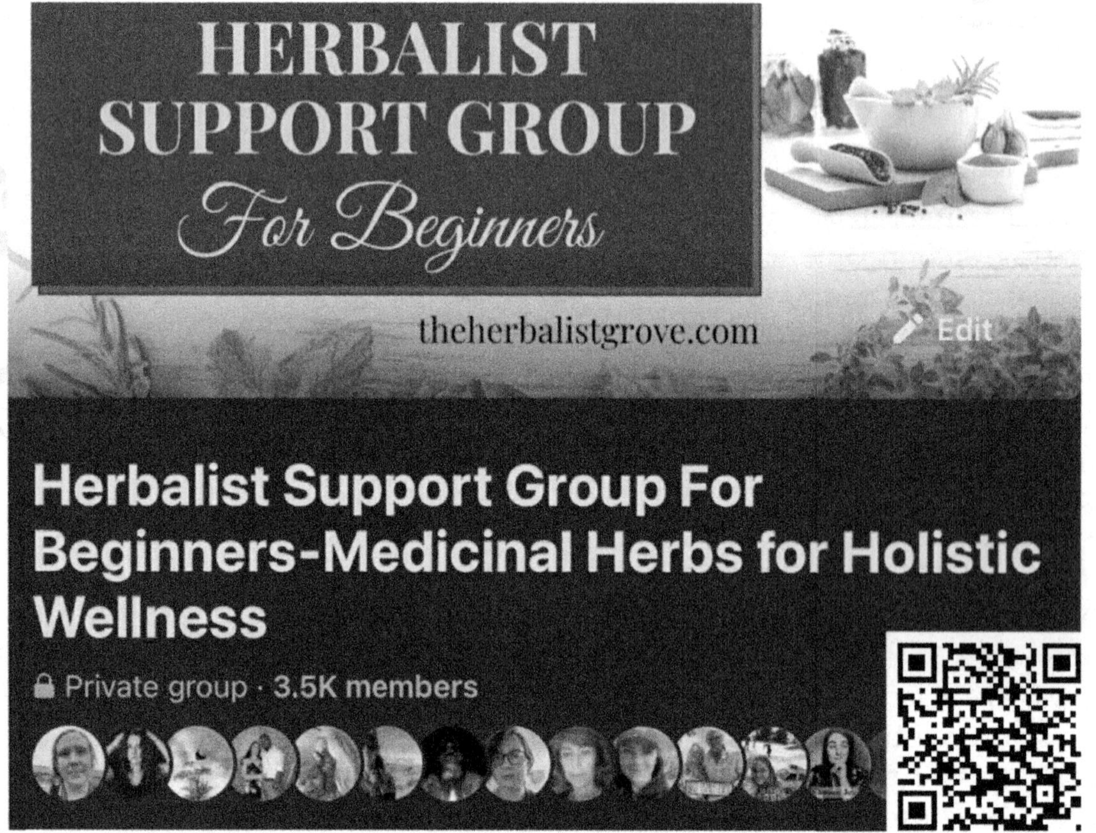

Connect with like-minded individuals in our private Facebook community!

GO TO Theherbalistgrove.com or
SCAN the QR code above to
JOIN NOW!

On Small Request...

As a self published auther, reviews are an enormous help! **It would mean the world to me** if you could leave a review. If you are enjoying this book so far... **please leave an Amazon review. It takes less than 30 seconds but means so much to me!**

Thank you and I can not wait to read your thoughts.

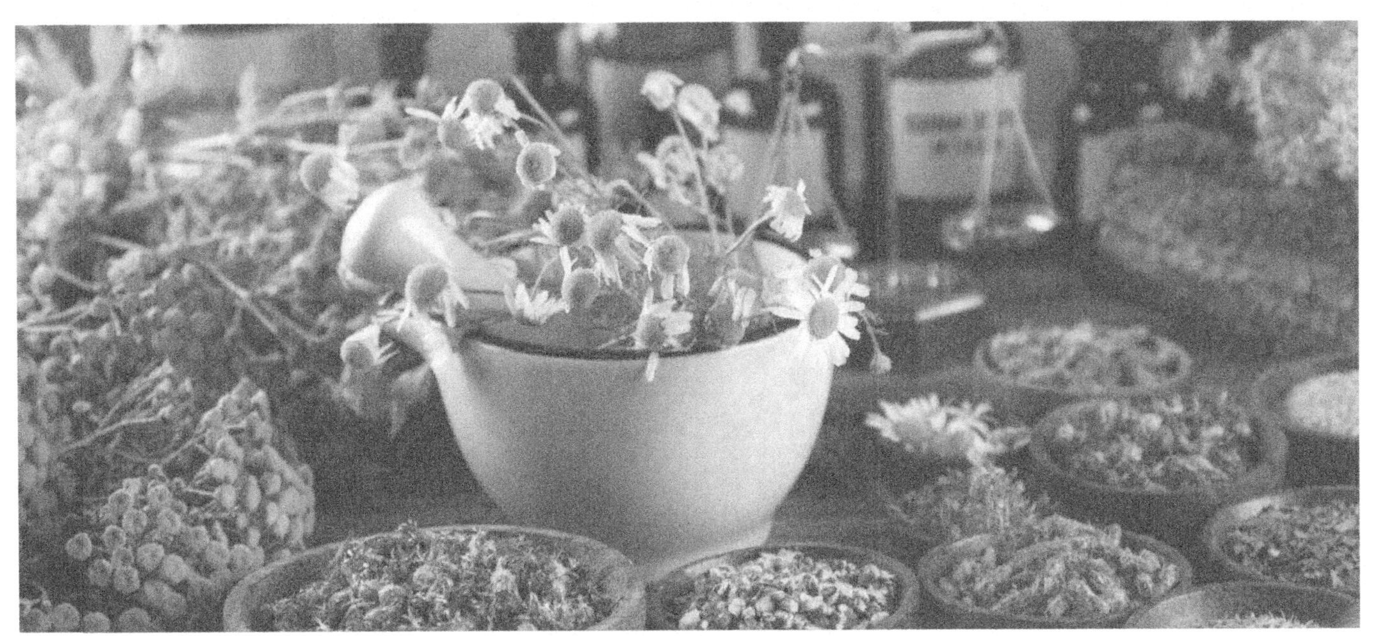

Chapter 6

26 Other Herbs to Have on Hand

Agrimony

Agrimonia eupatoria (Rosaceae)

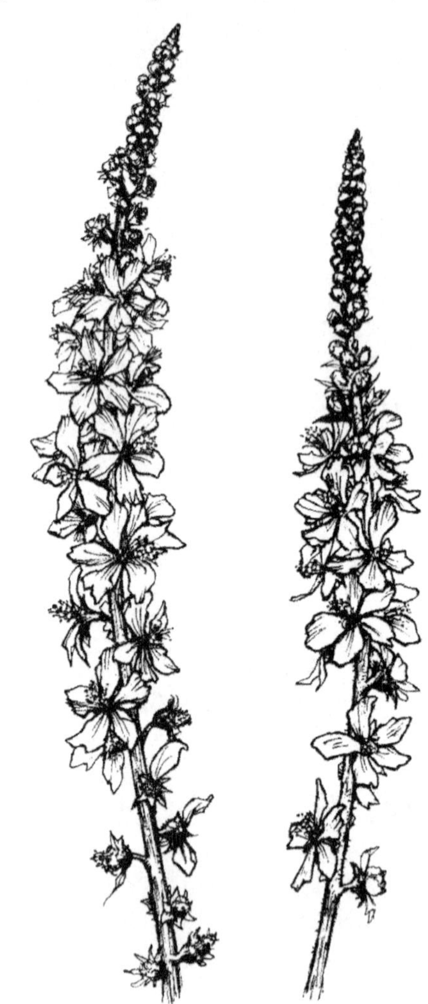

Agrimony, also referred to as liverwort or cocklebur, has beneficial anti-inflammatory properties. An infused tea of this fantastic herb may help improve digestion and lessen hyper-acidity. The tonic capacity of agrimony helps protect and strengthen the liver. This herbal action is vital because the liver performs over 500 functions in the body!

Description

Agrimony is a medium perennial plant belonging to the rose family. It can grow to 4 feet (120 centimeters) tall, with yellow flowers that are spiky and sprout from its long, pinnate stems. The alternate compound leaves bear tooth-like edges that yield a yellowish dye.

History

The initial idea about the herbal potential of agrimony was traced back to Northern Turkey's King of Pontus. During this time, common herbal preparations such as teas, tonics, and formulas were created for overall health. Also, the Anglo-Saxons taught that agrimony would heal snake bites, wounds, and warts during the early Middle Ages.

Habitat & Cultivation

Agrimony is native to European regions, but different varieties can grow in damp areas like wet meadows and marshes worldwide. This plant likes loamy, sandy, gravel, or silty soil and can thrive in full sunlight but does not mind partial shade. Agrimony flowers are essential in extracting this herb's active components. It is best to harvest the flowers from June to early September.

Active Compounds: Coumarin; Flavonoids; Polysaccharides; Tannins

Herbal Actions: Anti-inflammatory; Astringent; Tonic; Wound healing

Parts Used: Aerial parts

Main Use:

- Wound-healing agent because it can staunch bleeding and promote clot formation.
- May help individuals suffering from rheumatism and osteoarthritis.

Self-care Use:

- Diarrhea or general digestion issues
- Manage kidney stones
- Throat issues like sore throat and hoarseness

⚠ **Caution!**

- ★ Topical application of agrimony may cause the skin to become sensitive to sunlight.

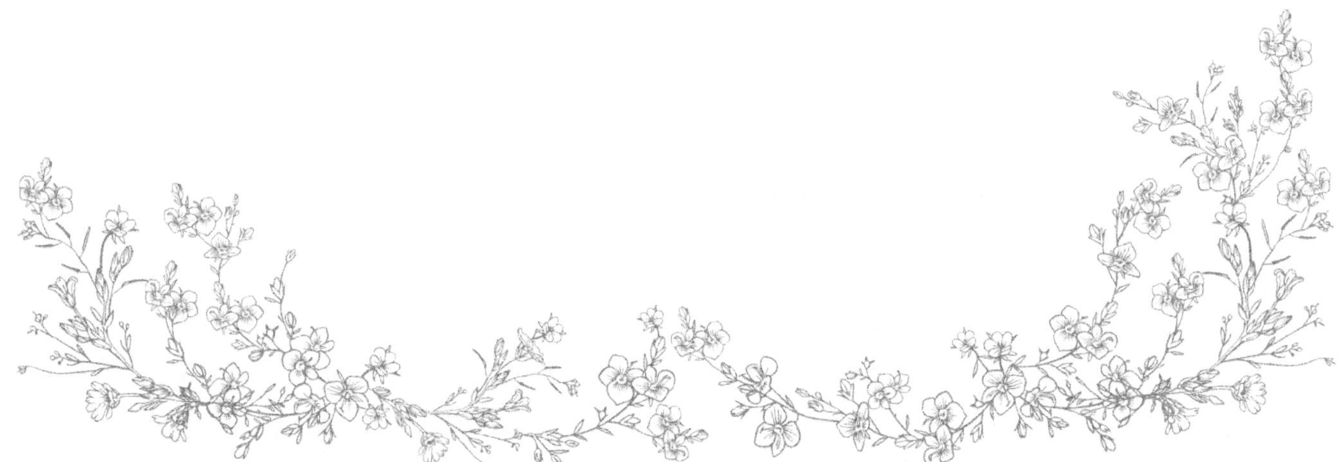

Aloe vera

Aloe vera syn. A. barbadensis (Xanthorrhoeaceae)

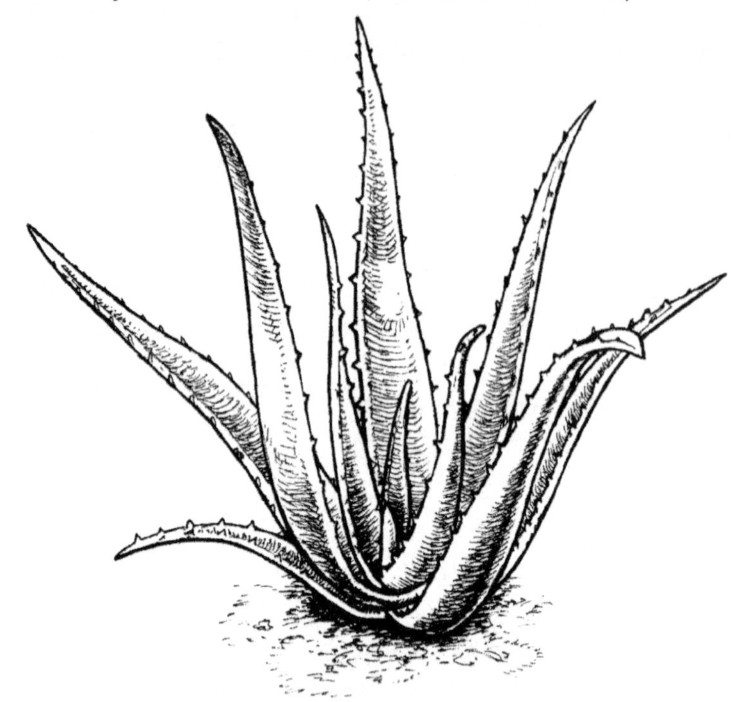

Aloe vera is one of the first plants that come to mind whenever I think about skincare. This prickly succulent contains a gel-like substance in its thick leaves that can manage wounds and burns but is also great for alleviating acne.

It is easy to use aloe vera in DIY herbal preparations to make a skincare regimen for topical applications. Just scoop the meat out of the leaves and blend it for a few minutes until frothy. You can also purchase aloe vera gels, ointments, or lotions at your local supermarkets.

Description

Aloe vera is a plant with virtually no stem and has very thick, fleshy leaves. If they do have a stem, it tends to be very short. The plant is generally stout and grows to about 2 feet (60.96 centimeters). Aloe vera's leaves vary in color from green to grayish with scattered white specks.

History

The Sumerians and Chinese had a record of using aloe vera as early as 3000 BC. Moreover, Egyptians also made great use of this fantastic plant. Cleopatra was one of the most iconic historical figures that regularly used aloe vera on her skin as a beauty treatment. Because of the versatility of aloe vera, Egyptian pharaohs crowned it as the "elixir of eternal life" *(Atalayabio, n.d.)*. Aloe veras' uses in the past are continuously being applied, cultivated, and studied by modern society.

Habitat & Cultivation

Aloe vera is found in most Mediterranean regions but is native to Northern and Eastern Africa. Because of its broad uses, it is globally cultivated. You can propagate aloe vera plants for home use by cutting a small plantlet and growing it in a pot. However, these potted aloe vera plants may have a lower anthraquinone content, a chemical component vital to its medicinal use. Your aloe plants will do best in temperatures between 55–80 °F (13–27 °C).

Active Compounds: Anthraquinones; Resins; Tannins; Polysaccharides; Aloectin B
Herbal Actions: Facilitates wound healing; Laxative; Stimulates the secretion of bile
Parts Used: Leaves
Main Use:

- Skincare soothes skin burns and bug bites.
- Constipation: The base of the leaves aids in bowel movement

Self-care Use:

- Soothes the skin and helps with minor burns and sunburn
- Stretch marks
- Warts, weeping skin, and wounds

⚠ **Caution!**

- ★ Avoid topically applying the bitter juice extracted from the base of the leaves.
- ★ Oral intake is not indicated for PREGNANT or breastfeeding women.
- ★ DO NOT take it if you have hemorrhoids or kidney disease.

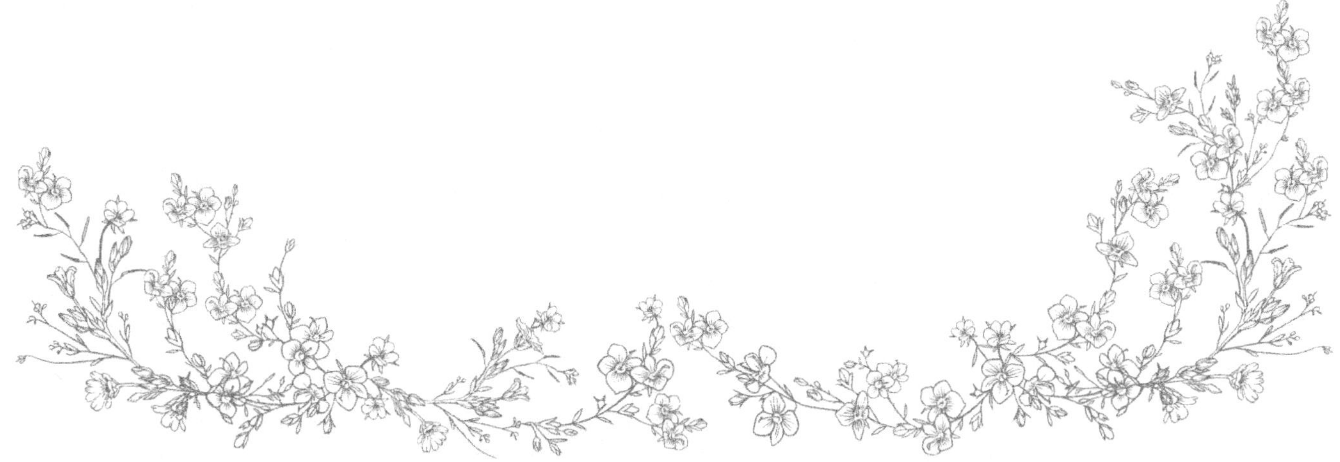

Angelica

Angelica archangelica (Apiaceae)

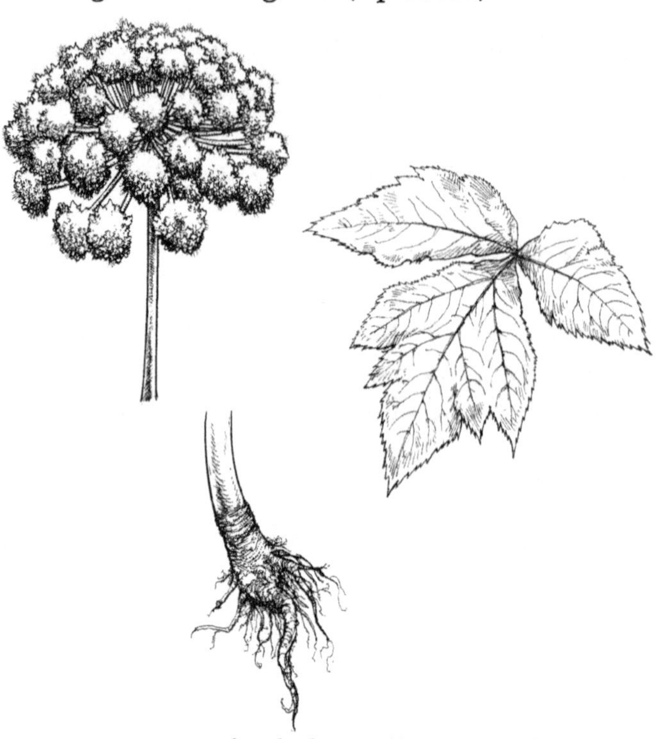

Asian countries have numerous herbal applications for angelica, including liver detoxification, blood circulation illnesses, and digestive ailments *(Shoemaker, 2020).* I use 1000 milligrams of angelica capsules for heartburn after eating spicy foods. It works every time! You can also use it in everyday cooking by adding it to soups, sautéing it as a side dish, or chopping it into fruit salads.

Description

Angelica is also called wild celery, and a mature angelica plant will grow to about 6.5 feet (2 meters) tall. Its ridged hollow stems are filled with numerous bipinnate leaves and greenish-white flowers. These flowers have compound umbels where many flower heads grow on one cluster.

History

Laplanders of the Viking society viewed angelica as one of their most essential plants. It is said that they used it to ease symptoms of colds, colic, digestive issues, and sore throats. During the era of Charles II, around the 1600s, angelica was used as a plague curative remedy *(Angelica, 2013).* The entire plant has been used in many herbal applications as well as for culinary purposes.

Habitat & Cultivation

The angelica herb prefers temperate areas such as those in the Himalayas, Western Europe, and Siberia. Damp locations help angelica thrive and obtain the optimum active components locked inside its parts. Harvest their leaves and stems in early summer, their seeds during late summer, and their roots in late autumn. Interestingly, angelica does not mature until it has been growing for two years, and in colder climates, it may take three to four years.

Active Compounds: Volatile oil (beta-phellandrene); Lactones; Coumarins
Herbal Actions: Anti-inflammatory; Tonic
Parts Used: All parts
Main Use:

- Can improve poor circulation and promote blood flow.
- The warm tonic capability can comfort bronchitis and respiratory problems.

Self-care Use:

- Alleviate stomach spasms
- Relieve gas, indigestion, and colic

⚠ **Caution!**

★ DO NOT take it if you are PREGNANT or plan to become pregnant.
★ DO NOT confuse it with Chinese Angelica.

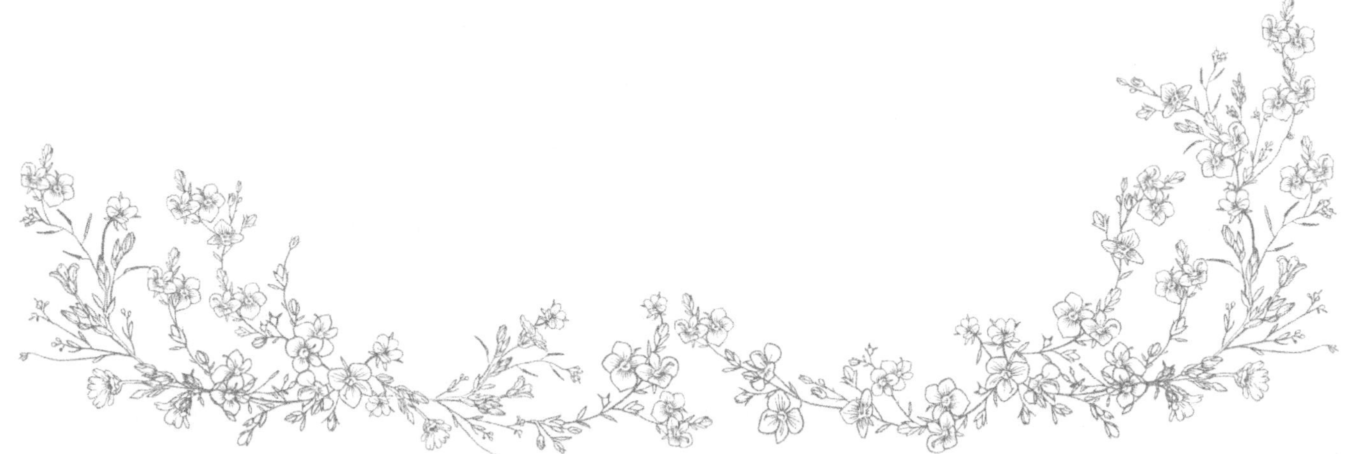

Bergamot

Citrus bergamia (Rutaceae)

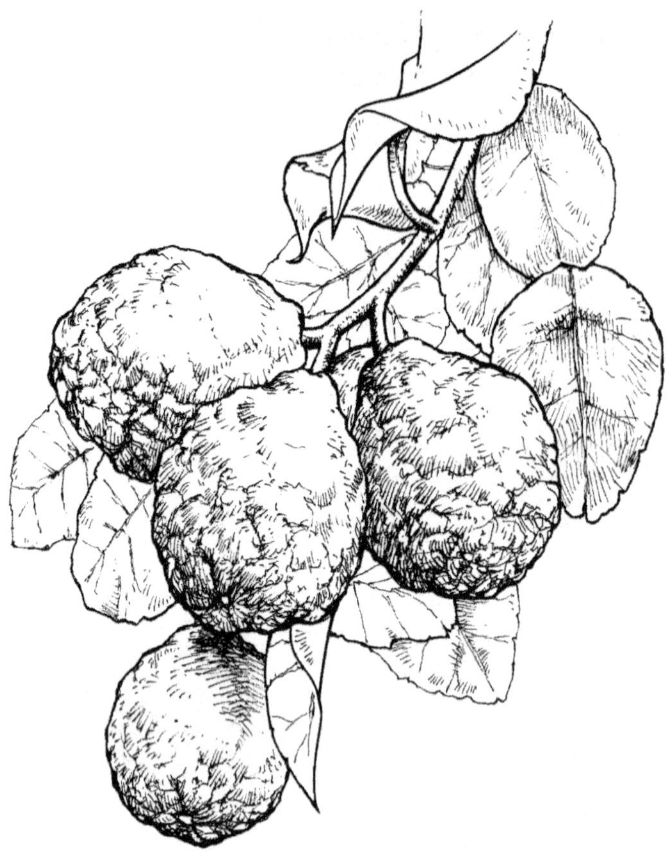

Bergamot trees produce small oranges from which essential oils are extracted from the peel *(Zielinski, 2021)*. The primary use for these essential oils is in aromatherapy. Aside from its calming fragrance, bergamot oil may relieve anxiety and can instantly enhance one's mood. I always have a bottle of bergamot essential oil next to my diffuser in my office to keep me focused and happy throughout busy workdays.

Description

Do not confuse the bergamot tree with the bergamot herb, also called bee balm. They are very different and come from entirely different plants. Bergamot is a tree that can grow up to 30 feet (10 meters) tall and spread its branches very wide. You can observe its pointy and ovate-shaped leaves with a light or dark green color. Its fruit and flowers have a uniquely enticing aroma with a citrusy and fruity scent.

History

Although there is not much information on the historical medicinal uses of this herb, it has been noted as a complementary and alternative therapy in Egypt, India, and China for nearly 6000 years *(Maruca, 2017)*. This documentation was the beginning of bergamot's aromatherapy applications. It is one of the only citrus essential oils used in aromatherapy that calms the nervous system rather than stimulates it.

Bergamot also has an exciting history in the cosmetic and perfume industries. The first recorded account of it being used as a fragrance was in 1714 in a perfume made by a German woman named Jean-Marie Farina. She called it *Eau de Cologne*, meaning "water from Cologne," a city in Germany. Cologne has since become the standard term for scented formulations.

Habitat & Cultivation

Bergamot orange trees are native to tropical Asia but are almost exclusively cultivated on the coastal plains of southern Italy. They can be planted outdoors in regions with very mild winters. If your climate allows, be sure to plant your tree in well-endowed sunlight to ensure the growth of your bergamot oranges.

Active Compounds: Volatile oils – Linalyl acetate (30–60%), Limonene (26–42%), Linalool (11–22%); Bergapten; Diterpene

Herbal Actions: Soothing agent; Anti-inflammatory; Antioxidant; Antibacterial

Parts Used: Flowers; Essential oil from the peel of the fruit

Main Use:

- Topically applied as palliative care to external conditions
- Essential oils may soothe skin irritations like eczema, hives, and psoriasis

Self-care Use:

- Can be topically applied to bring relief to tense or spasmodic muscles and improve digestion

⚠ Caution!

★ Bergamot oil should NOT be taken internally.

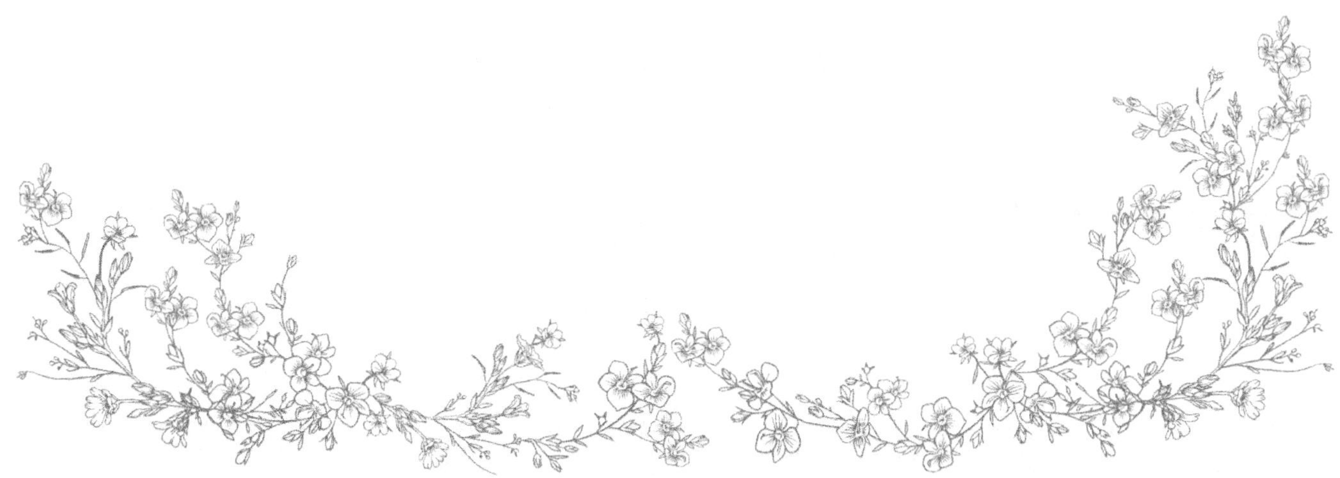

Buckwheat

Fagopyrum esculentum (Polygonaceae)

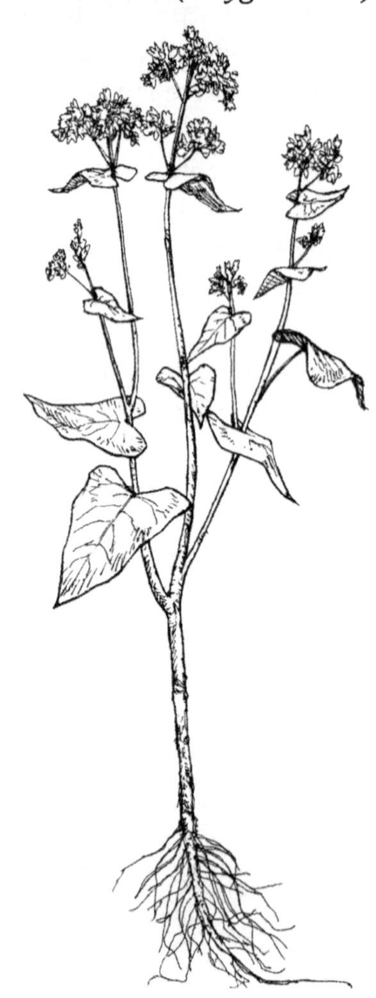

Despite having "wheat" in its name, and consumption as a cereal grain, buckwheat is a pseudo-cereal. The benefits of this plant include high antioxidant content, fiber, protein, and minerals. Aside from this, buckwheat may also be vital for different heart and blood vessel ailments. If you want a more holistic approach to diabetes, high cholesterol, heart disease, and varicose veins, then buckwheat might just be the plant you need.

Description

Buckwheat is an annual that grows up to 20 inches (50 centimeters) tall. The leaves of this plant have a unique heart shape and have clustered white or pink flowers. It has stems that are hollow and reddish. Buckwheat seeds are triangular and encased in a dark brown rind.

History

Buckwheat originated from the ancient Middle East but eventually was carried to Europe during the 11th-century Crusades. Other historians argued that it might be the other way around. The Spaniards might have brought buckwheat into the Arab regions *(Perez, 2018).* Practical applications of buckwheat in Traditional Chinese Medicine (TCM) have been used for centuries to aid ailments such as ulcers and hypertension.

Habitat & Cultivation

Buckwheat is native to Tibet, China, and the Eastern Himalayas. This herb thrives in the northern hemisphere and is harvested in Russia, China, Europe, and Kazakhstan. Unfortunately, buckwheat would not succeed in scorching and dry climates. It is best to sow its seeds from late spring to summer. This plant enjoys well-balanced soil and full to partial shade.

Active Compounds: Bioflavonoids (rutin)

Herbal Actions: Antioxidants

Parts Used: Leaves, Flowers, Seeds

Main Use:

- Used for circulatory ailments.

Self-care Use:

- Its tea or tablet can be used in helping manage high blood pressure and arteriosclerosis.

⚠ **Caution!**

- ★ Avoid buckwheat if you are taking blood-thinning medications and anticoagulants because it may interfere with its actions

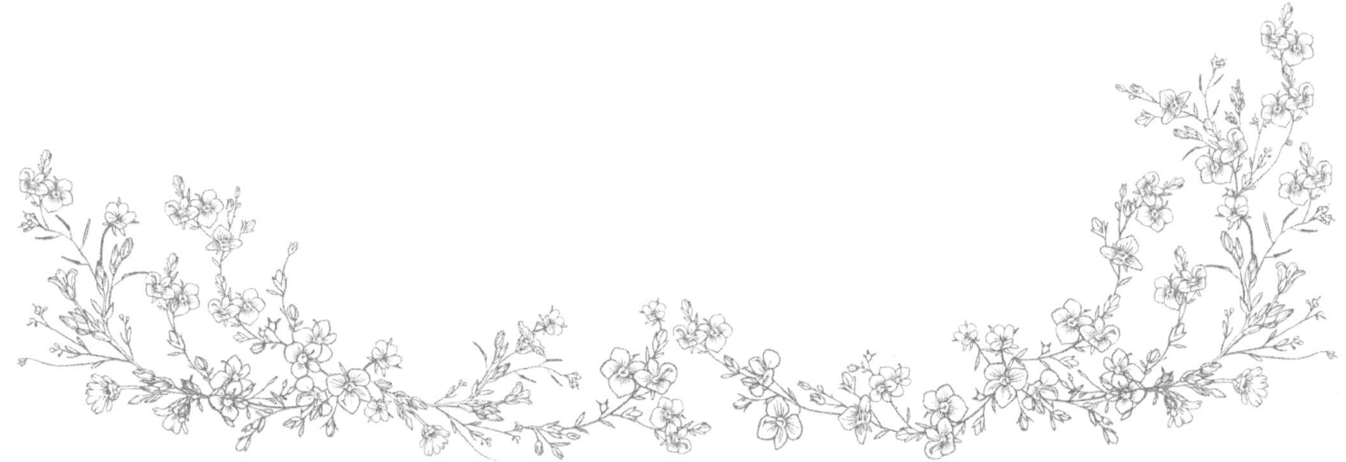

Calendula

Calendula officinalis (Asteraceae)

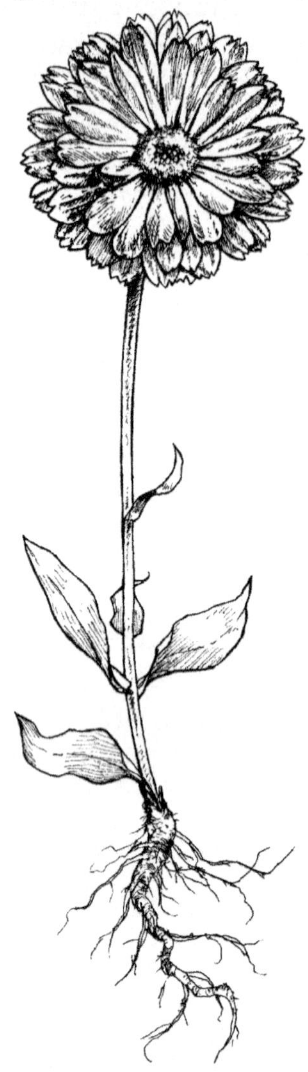

Studies show that the high levels of carotenoids and flavonoids in calendula could help reverse cancer and heart disease *(Lang, 2020)*. Calendula is known for its antioxidant and anti-inflammatory properties and may help prevent infections and injury. When I have sore muscles, I reach for this remarkable herb. Applying a calendula poultice to the affected area has a soothing effect that decreases inflammation and allows my body to heal naturally.

Description

Calendula can grow to almost 2 feet (nearly 61 cemeteries) tall and displays very vibrant yellow to orange-colored flowers. A notable identifying factor is its smooth and waxy stems. The leaves are typically toothed along the edges; some varieties have no stalk between the leaf and stem.

History

Ancient Romans noticed that this herb bloomed like clockwork every first day of the month, so they named it calendula, which means "little clock" in Latin *(Fischer, 2020)*. They utilized this plant in rituals by making the flowers into crowns. Aztecs, Mayans, and Catholics used calendula for their ancient ceremonies. It was also prominent in herbalism as an antiseptic and disinfectant.

During the Civil War and again during World War I, calendula was documented as a great herb to help control bleeding in wounded soldiers.

Calendula is also called marigold, based on an early church legend. As the story goes, when Mary and Joseph fled to Egypt, robbers stole Mary's purse. They were surprised to find it filled with golden flowers. From then on, calendula was known as "Mary's Gold."

Habitat & Cultivation

Calendula is native to the temperate climates of Southern Europe and Northern Africa, but you can grow this wonderful herb at home if you have the right conditions. This herb is commonly called pot marigold; as the name implies, they love to be cultivated in pots. They can be grown in the ground with nutrient-rich organic soil and plenty of space to grow. You can harvest the flowers during early summer and utilize them in your herbal apothecary.

Active Compounds: Bitter glycosides; Carotenes; Flavonoids; Resins; Triterpenes; Volatile oil

Herbal Actions: Anti-inflammatory; Antimicrobial; Astringent; Detoxifying; Mild estrogenic; Relieves muscles spasm; Wound healing

Parts Used: Flowers (dried or fresh)

Main Use:

- Managing bleeding and healing in small cuts/scrapes
- Managing fungal infections: athlete's foot, thrush, and ringworm.

Self-care Use:

- Effective on minor skin issues: soothing diaper rash, inflamed skin, hives, acne and boils, and varicose veins.
- Infusion or tinctures for gastritis or peptic ulcers.
- Soothe breast tenderness and sore nipples

⚠ **Caution!**

- ★ DO NOT take if you are PREGNANT
- ★ DO NOT take if you are taking other sedatives or medications for blood pressure management

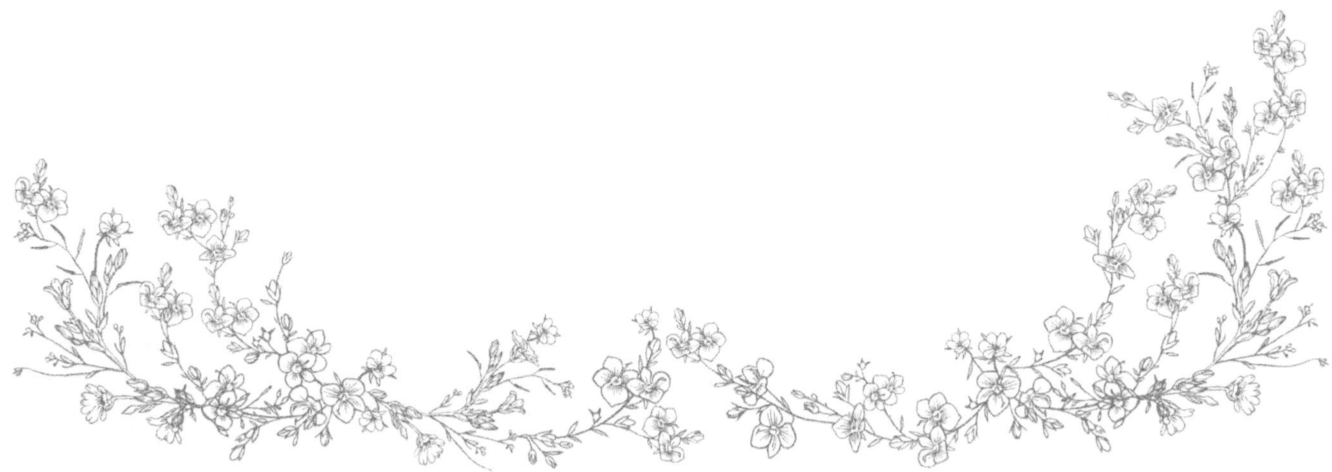

Comfrey

Symphytum officinale (Boraginaceae)

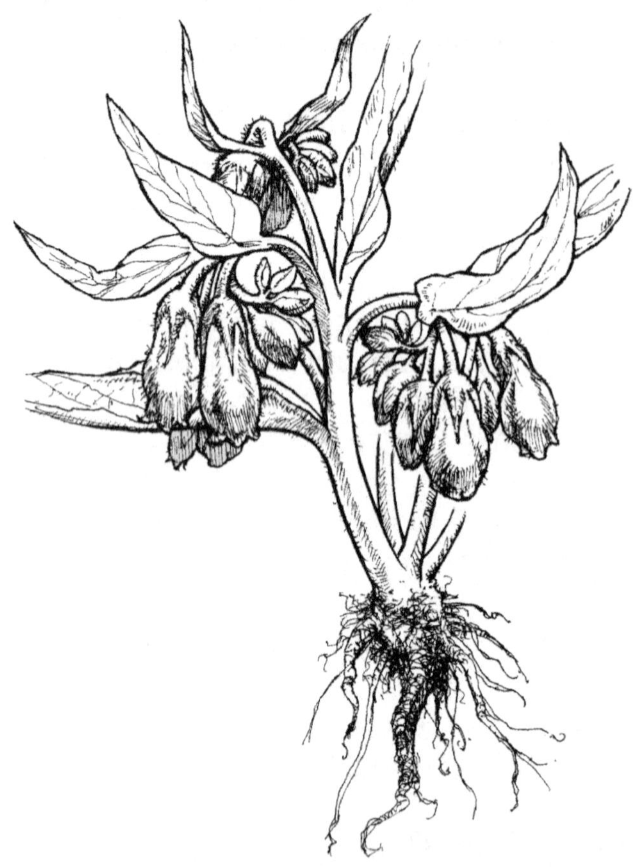

Different societies use the roots and leaves of comfrey topically for sprains, burns, inflammation, and even as a poultice for stomach ailments. I am naturally clumsy, and comfrey has been my go-to topical aid for bruises and swelling. I am what they call an accident-prone person, and while hiking, I often roll my ankles. I apply my homemade comfrey cream to the affected area, wait about 10 minutes, and then I am back up and ready to go.

Description

Comfrey can grow to about 3 feet (1 meter) high and about 30 inches (76 centimeters) wide. This shrub has drooping clusters of pink-purple bell-shaped flowers and ovate-shaped fuzzy leaves. The roots are slender and black-skinned.

History

Comfrey has been cultivated since about 400 BC. The name comes from the Latin "grow together." For this reason, the Greeks and Romans used it as a herbal aid for broken bones, wound healing, bronchial issues, and to stop heavy bleeding. Although this herb is native to Britain, English immigrants brought wild comfrey to the United States.

Habitat & Cultivation

As long as the climate is temperate, expect comfrey to thrive. These plants are indigenous to Europe but grow in moist and damp areas worldwide. If you cultivate this plant at home, you may want to grow it in a container or pot because it can be invasive once established. You can sow its seeds during spring, but it also propagates well from a cutting. Make sure to plant it in full to partial sun in a loamy soil.

Active Compounds: Allantoin; Asparagine; Mucilage; Phenolic acids; Pyrrolizidine alkaloids; Tannins; Triterpenoids

Herbal Actions: Anti-inflammatory; Astringent; Demulcent; Wound and bone healing

Parts Used: Root (fresh or dried); Aerial parts

Main Use:

- Traditionally used for healing sprains and fractures.

Self-care Use:

- Topically: skin inflammation, insect bites, and acne
- Poultice or ointment for fractures and bruises

⚠ **Caution!**

- ★ Avoid applying on dirty wounds to avoid microorganisms from invading the healing site.
- ★ Avoid using comfrey if you are PREGNANT or breastfeeding.
- ★ ☠ Comfrey for internal use has been connected to liver damage, liver cancer, mutagenicity, and even death. Only take internally for a short period of time and under the supervision of a professional.

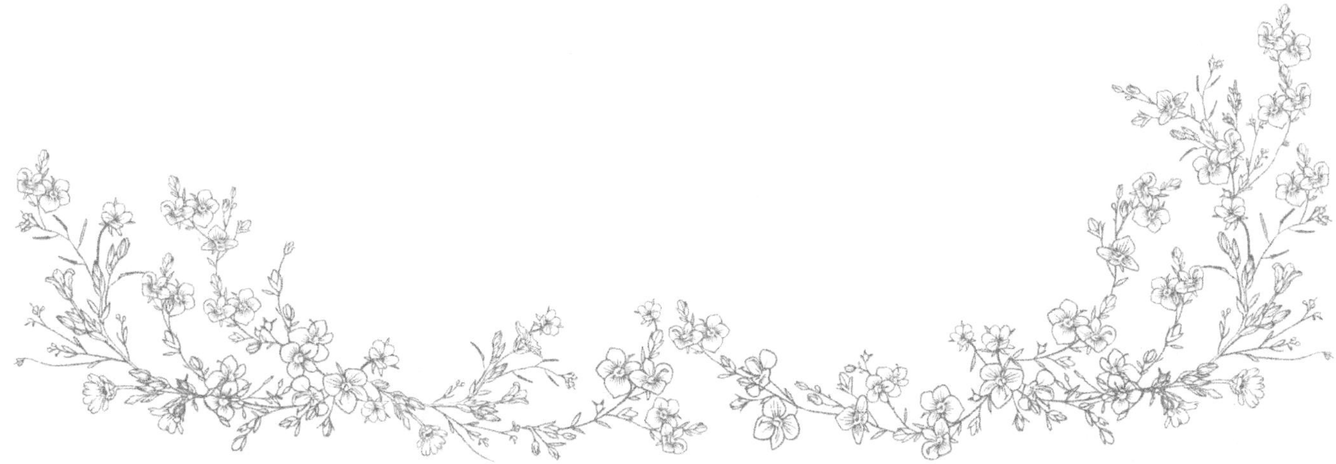

Chickweed

Stellaria media (Caryophyllaceae)

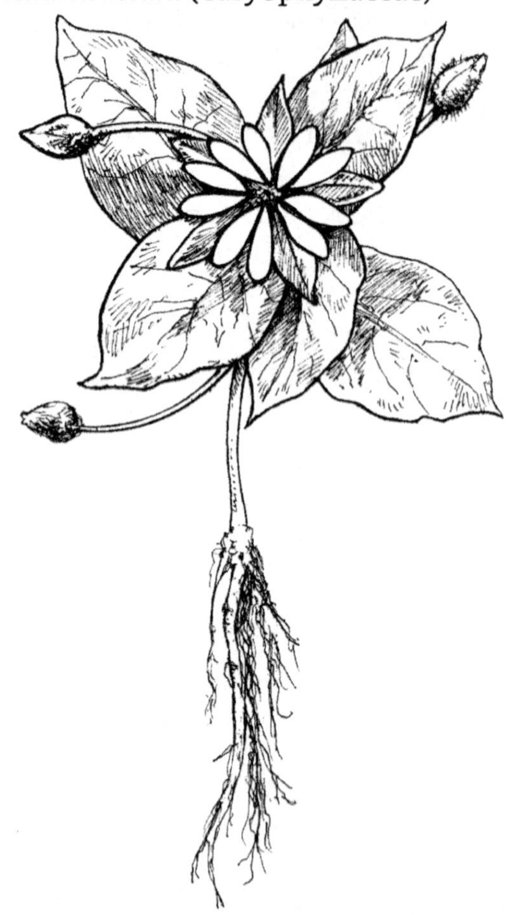

Chickweed is a versatile herb used for a myriad of ailments. You can ingest it raw for asthma, lung issues, constipation, and stomach problems. I particularly like to use chickweed ointments for my eczema. The active compounds in this herb help calm inflammation and reduce itchiness. It is also packed with many minerals and vitamins, including a high quantity of iron. For this reason, many people reach for chickweed to alleviate anemia.

Description

Chickweed is an annual plant but can grow all year long, even after it goes to seed. It has slender hairy stems that reach about 0.5–1 inch (1.27–2.54 centimeters) long and crawl along the ground. Their flowers are white and have a unique star-shaped appearance, while the leaves are ovate and smooth along the edges.

History

The Ancient Greeks had many applications for chickweed during the 1st century AD. Dioscorides, noted chickweed mixed with cornmeal and applied topically, would lessen eye inflammation, while its juice would help earaches *(Hunter, 2010)*. Even Ancient European sailors thought of chickweed as a valuable medicinal herb. They used it as a treatment for scurvy when citrus was not available.

Habitat & Cultivation

Chickweed is native to regions of Asia and Europe. Today, expect to see it growing in numerous parts of the world because it is effortless to grow and cultivate. It prefers neutral soil and dislikes acid soil conditions. Interestingly, some individuals see chickweed as an invasive and harmful weed.

Active Compounds: Carboxylic acid; Coumarins; Flavonoids; Saponins; Triterpenoid; Vitamin C

Herbal Actions: Anti-inflammatory

Parts Used: Aerial parts

Main Use:

- Mainly used as an anti-inflammatory agent.

Self-care Use:

- Topical preparation for joint inflammation, eczema, or hives.
- Reduces itchiness

⚠ **Caution!**

- ★ DO NOT take it if you are PREGNANT.
- ★ Large doses may lead to diarrhea and vomiting.

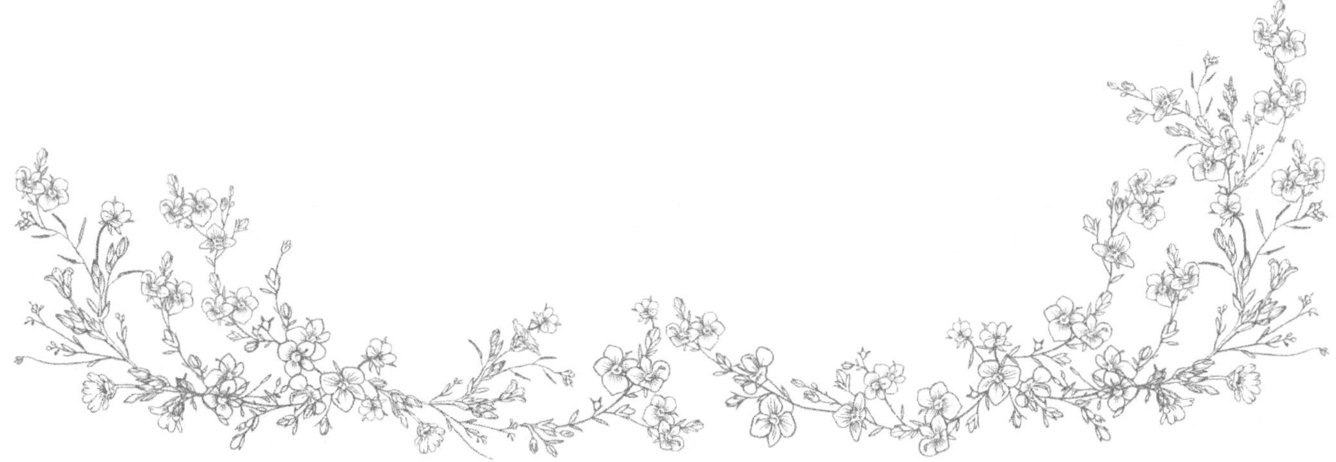

Dandelion

Taraxacum officinale (Asteraceae)

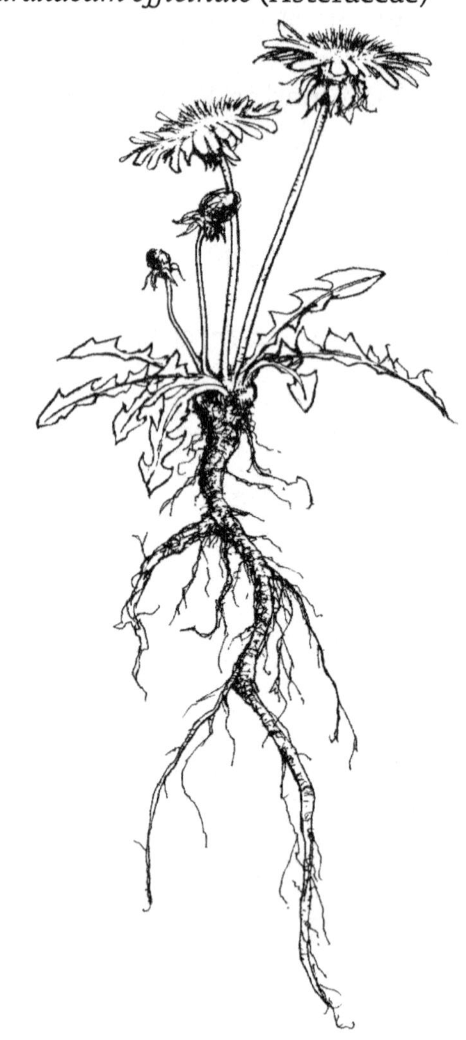

Although some might look at dandelions and think of them as pesky weeds, this herb has to be one of my all-time favorites. The entire plant is edible and can be used for many applications. It is a hardy plant I keep on hand, whether adding a handful of leaves to a salad to boost my immune system or brewing a cup of detoxifying dandelion root tea.

Description

Dandelion plants are herbaceous perennials that can easily be identified by their bright yellow flowers and deeply toothed basal leaves (leaves that only grow from the bottom of the stem). These leaves emerge from the crown at ground level and are connected to the taproot. The plant can grow from 2–24 inches (5.08–60.96 centimeters) tall with stems that do not branch and are hollow. If the leaves or stems are damaged, they will ooze a milky sap.

History

Dandelions have been used throughout the ages for their medicinal properties. They were named from the French term referring to a "lion's tooth" *(Caron, 2021)*. Traditional Chinese Medicine has used this powerful plant for over a thousand years to treat inflammation and stomach ailments. In the early 11th century, Arab physicians recommended this plant as a diuretic and an aid in maintaining liver health. When the Europeans traveled to the Americas in the mid-1600s, they brought dandelions to cultivate for food and medicine.

Habitat & Cultivation

At one time, this plant was mainly cultivated in Germany and France, but now dandelions are prevalent and can be found growing in most parts of the world. If you have seen a dandelion going to seed, you know how easily its seeds spread.

If you prefer to have this wonderful herb on hand, you can germinate its seeds for 7–21 days. They grow fast, and the flowers mature within 9–15 days. The entire plant can be harvested during the spring for optimum benefits.

Active Compounds: Polysaccharides; Sesquiterpene lactones; Triterpenes

Herbal Actions: Bitter; Detoxifying; Diuretic

Parts Used: All parts

Main Use:

- Diuretic
- High blood pressure

Self-care Use:

- Decoction, tincture, or juice: gut health and liver detoxification
- Roots can be made into a decoction for constipation.

⚠ **Caution!**

★ Can interact with other medications you are currently taking, such as diuretics.

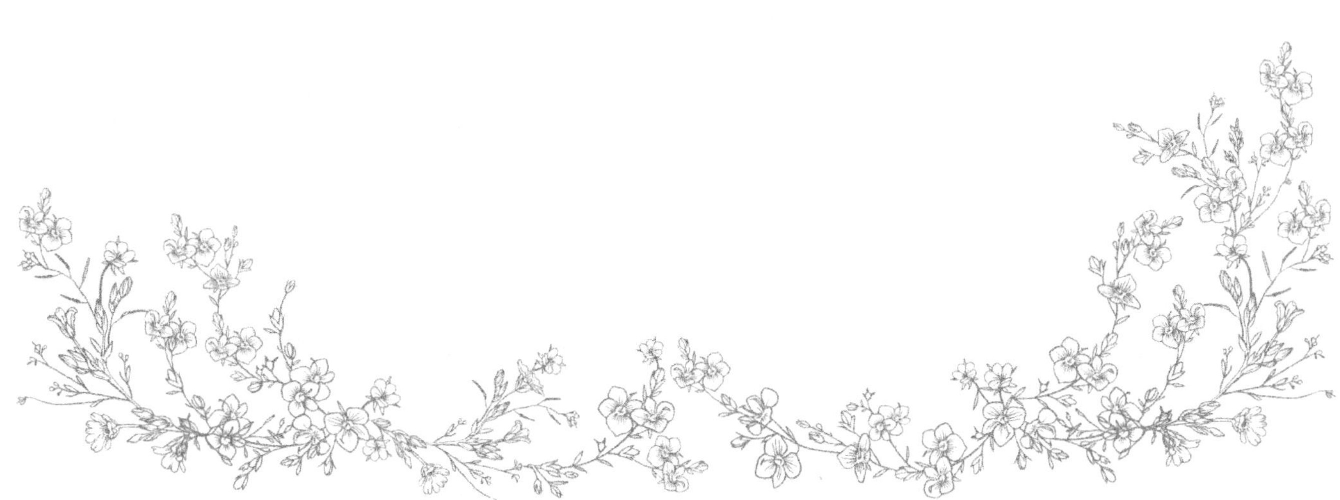

Echinacea

Echinacea spp. (Asteraceae)

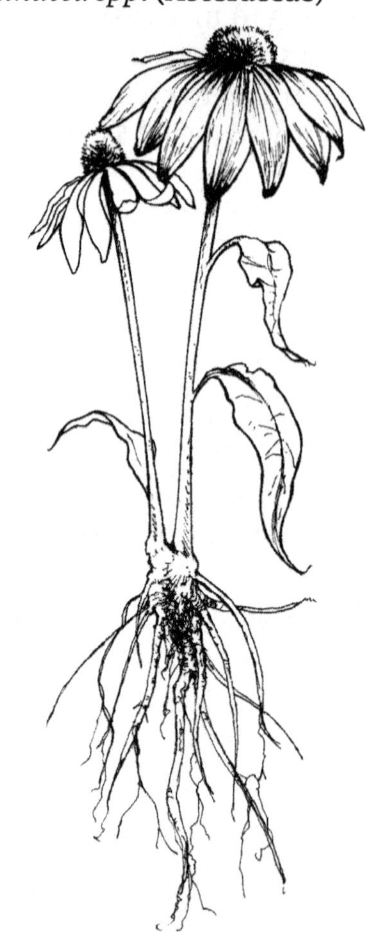

One of the most common herbal products for colds and flu is echinacea. Over-the-counter herbal products made from this herb are extensive since they are practical and well-tolerated. A sore throat can get uncomfortable, but lucky for me, a quick swish of an echinacea root decoction helps me feel better and eliminates the irritation.

Description

Echinacea is a perennial coneflower that grows up to 4 feet (140 centimeters) tall, depending on the species, and is adorned with a single purple-pink flower. The cone in the center is typically purple or brownish colored. The stems are slender, and their leaves have a rough texture.

History

Echinacea has been used for centuries by Native Americans for a variety of ailments, including colds and toothaches. It was nicknamed Indian Snakeroot because of its ability to remove toxins caused by snake bites. It was not until the 19th century that the pharmaceutical science of this plant was explored, and by 1939 commercial cultivation began in Germany.

Habitat & Cultivation

Native to North America, these plants grow in open and wooded areas. ALL species of echinacea have become threatened by overharvesting in the wild. Therefore you should ONLY purchase commercially grown plants or propagate from seed. Plant them in nutrient-rich sandy soil and full to partial sun.

Active Compounds: Alkylamides; Caffeic acid esters; Polysaccharides
Herbal Actions: Anti-inflammatory; Antimicrobial; Antioxidant; Stimulates salivation; Wound healing
Parts Used: Flowers and Roots
Main Use:

- Alleviate toothache or throat infections
- Wound-healing ability and antimicrobial effects on rabies and snake bites

Self-care Use:

- Manage skin infections like boils, acne, and fungal infections
- Soothe bites and stings

⚠ **Caution!**

- ★ Can be an allergen

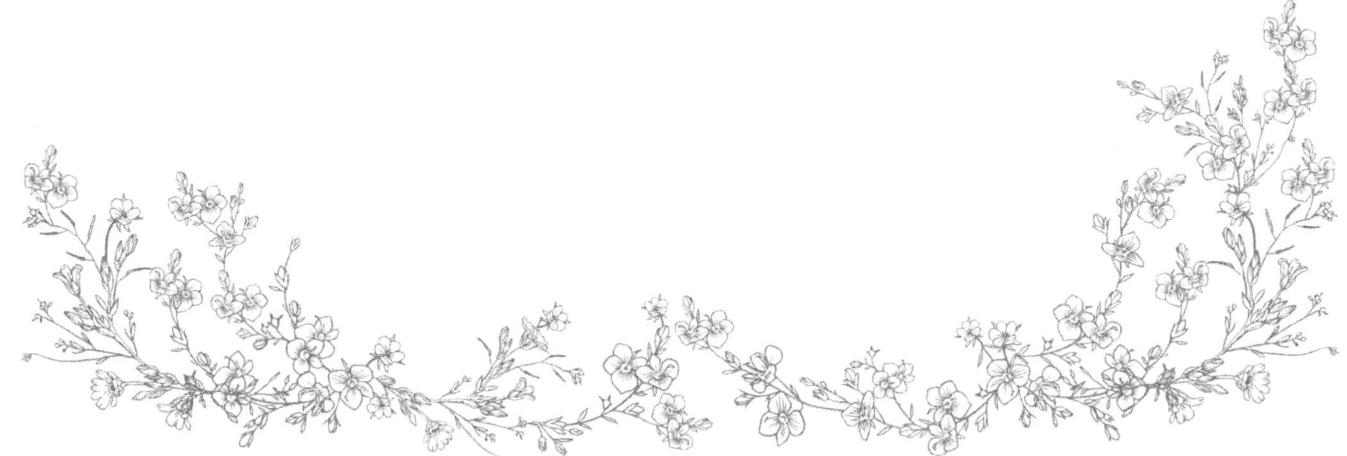

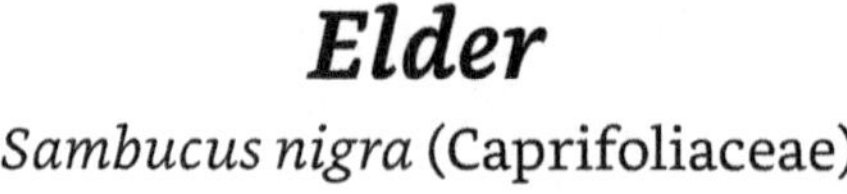

Elder

Sambucus nigra (Caprifoliaceae)

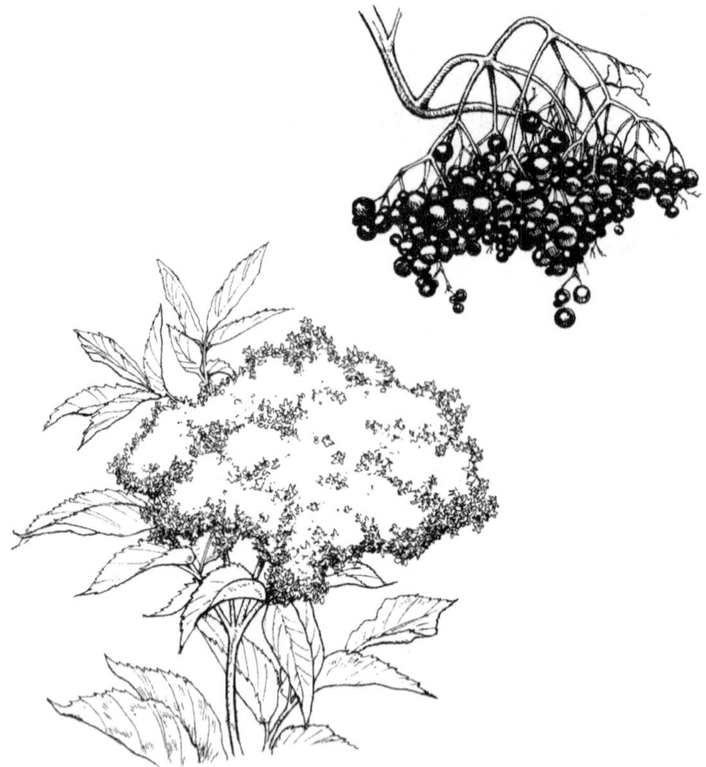

Elder is used as a handy herb for combatting and relieving different ailments. Sometimes, we cannot avoid catching a cold. With elder tea, alleviating a runny nose, allergies, and even flu symptoms is easy. The leaves may aid in healing bruises, while the flowers are great for sinus issues, and the berries can help boost your immune system.

Description

Ten species of elders vary in size, from short shrubs to tall trees. The elder *Sambucus nigra* is a deciduous tree that can grow between about 9–30 feet (3–10 meters) tall and equally wide. It has a gray bark that changes to a darker tone, indicating the tree's age. Each tree leaf contains five to seven leaflets with toothed edges and pointy tips. You can also identify the tree by its white flowers and small dark purple berries.

History

Elder has a rich history dating back to around 2000 BC. During this time, they discovered seeds from the tree in Neolithic pole-dwellings in Switzerland. The plant received its name during the Greco-Roman period, and many Greek herbal scholars wrote of its medicinal properties. Even Dioscorides wrote about it in his *Materia Medica.*

Being dubbed “nature’s medicine chest,” elders have rich folklore showing how much value the early English society put on this tree. The tale describes that the nymph goddess of vegetation, Hylde Moer, lived in the elder tree and chopping the branches without asking was considered dangerous *(Brobst, 2013)*. If one did not recite a prayer before taking from the elder, Hylde Moer would set a plague upon them.

Habitat & Cultivation

This particular elder is native to Europe, Africa, and Southwest Asia, where you can find it growing wild. If you want to try cultivating trees at home, you can expect to see them grow 2–3 feet in the first year. Although they prefer moist, well-draining soil, they can adapt to other grounds. Keep them in full sunlight, and they will thrive.

Active Compounds: Anthocyanins; Flavonoids; Lectins; Mucilage; Tannins; Triterpenes; Vitamins A and C; Volatile Oil

Herbal Actions: Anti-inflammatory; Antiviral; Diuretic; Expectorant; Perspirant

Parts Used: Flowers; Berries; Leaves

Main Use:

- Colds, flu, coughs, and other upper respiratory tract infections
- Sinus decongestant and alleviates throat itchiness

Self-care Use:

- Flower infusions: colds
- Berries: arthritis
- Mild laxative
- May lower blood pressure

⚠ **Caution!**

★ It is recommended to avoid eating unripe berries.

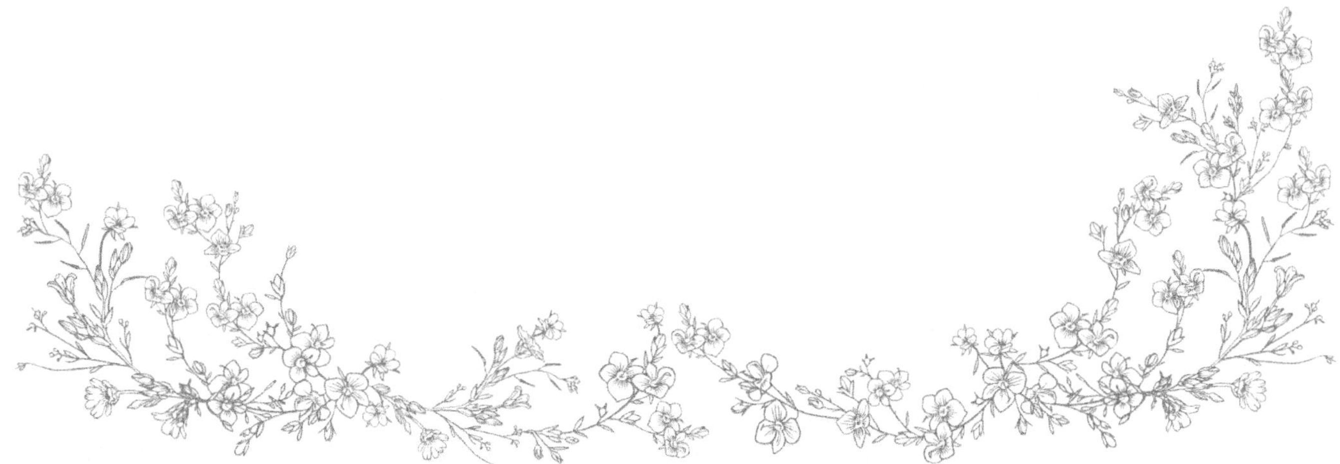

Fennel

Foeniculum vulgare (Apiaceae)

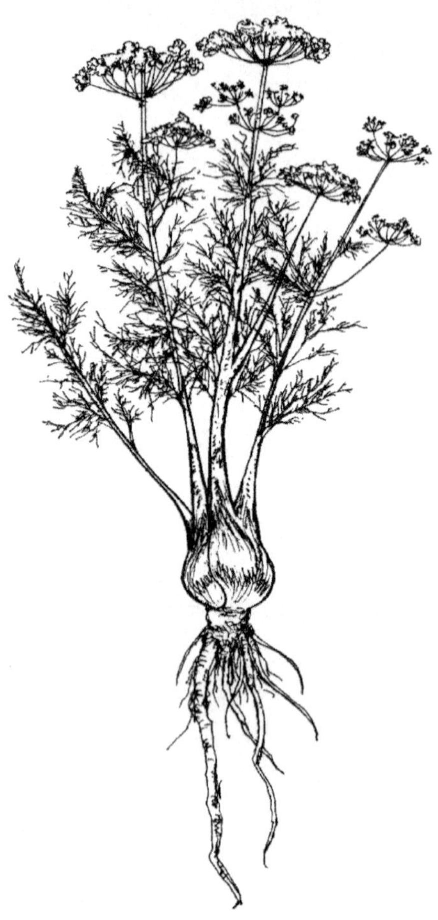

Fennel seeds are the most utilized part of this plant as these provide a robust flavor and added medicinal properties. Some evidence-based advantages of fennel include better heart health, reduced cancer risk, and benefits for breastfeeding mothers (Kubala, 2019). The entire plant is edible and provides the body with essential nutrients, including fiber and potassium.

Description

Fennel is an aromatic plant that grows from a bulb and reaches up to 5 feet (1.5 meters) tall. When fennel plants cluster together, their dark green leaves appear feathery. This plant is adorned with small yellow flowers and presents a licorice-like aroma and taste. Do not worry! The licorice taste lessens when cooked, and even licorice haters enjoy fennel.

History

Throughout history, ancient societies used fennel as both food and medicine. The Chinese have been using it for centuries for snake bites. Even Dioscorides recorded his 1st-century use of fennel juice in the eyes for better vision and putting it into infected ears as an antimicrobial agent.

Habitat & Cultivation

Fennel is native to temperate regions of the Mediterranean. Generally, a mild climate is suitable for this plant's growth. If you want to grow fennel at home, use raised garden beds or well-draining containers to prevent root rot. You can grow from seed, but once the seedlings are easy to handle, thin them out to about 12 inches apart to give them space to grow. Harvest your fennel seeds during autumn for the highest quality.

Active Compounds: Coumarins; Flavonoids; Sterol; Vitamins A, C, and B6; Volatile oils
Herbal Actions: Anti-inflammatory; Antispasmodic; Bitter
Parts Used: Seeds, Aerial parts, Bulb
Main Use:

- Stomach pain and inflammation
- Diuretic: urinary infections or kidney stones

Self-care Use:

- Gargle for sore throats
- Increases production of breastmilk in lactating mothers.
- Essential oils: relieve digestive ailments and alleviate stress and anxiety

⚠ **Caution!**

- ★ May be toxic if excessive doses are taken ☠
- ★ DO NOT take essential oils internally.

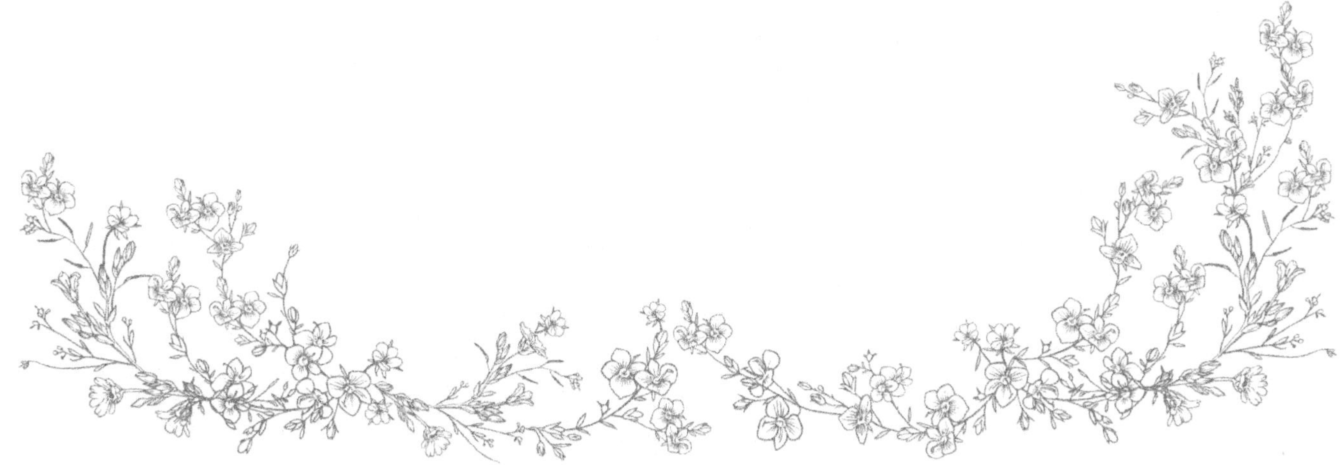

Feverfew

Tanacetum parthenium (Asteraceae)

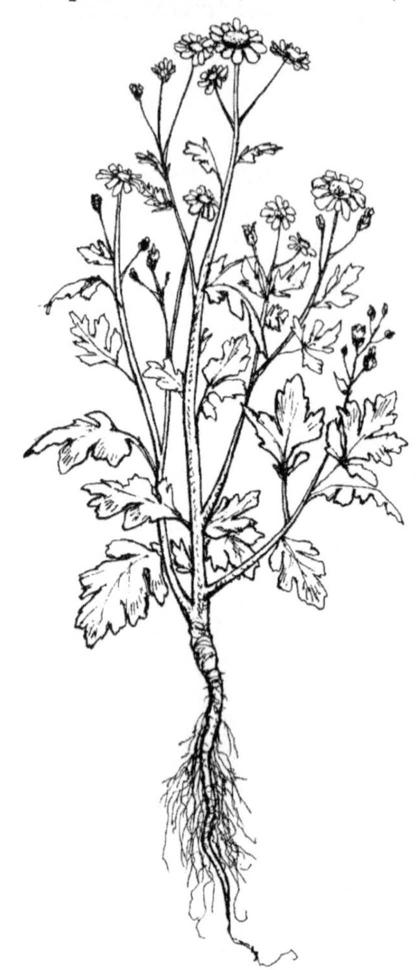

One of many uses of feverfew is relieving and managing migraines' symptoms. My mother swears by this powerful herb and takes it anytime she feels that throbbing feeling in her temples trying to take hold. You can easily make a feverfew tincture, brew an herbal tea, or purchase supplements at your local drug store.

Description

Feverfew is a flowering shrub adorned with small white flowers with yellow centers, similar to daisies. The stems are noted to have a light green color which may be angular or longitudinally furrowed. These stems can grow from 8–24 inches (20.32–60.96 centimeters) tall with yellow-green hairy leaves.

History

Feverfew came from "febrifugia," a Latin word that means reducing fever *(Raman, 2019).* Its predominant use in the 1st century BC was to decrease fevers and most inflammatory conditions. Also, women thoroughly benefited from feverfew during the 1600s. Traditionally, it was an herb that cleansed and strengthened a woman's womb.

Habitat & Cultivation

Feverfew is now commonly growing in most parts of Europe, North America, and Australia. You can quickly cultivate the seeds and cuttings in well-draining soil with plenty of sunlight. Most aerial parts benefit our health and are best harvested during summer – the season where its flowers bloom.

Active Compounds: Camphor; Parthenolide; Volatile oil

Herbal Actions: Analgesic; Anti-inflammatory; Anti-rheumatic; Diuretic; Promotes menstrual flow; Reduces fever

Parts Used: Flower and leaves

Main Use:

- Migraine and headaches

Self-care Use:

- Reduce fevers
- Arthritis

⚠ **Caution!**

★ May interfere with medications like blood thinners.
★ Consuming fresh feverfew leaves can lead to mouth ulcers.
★ Taken in large quantities: may cause abdominal pain and diarrhea.

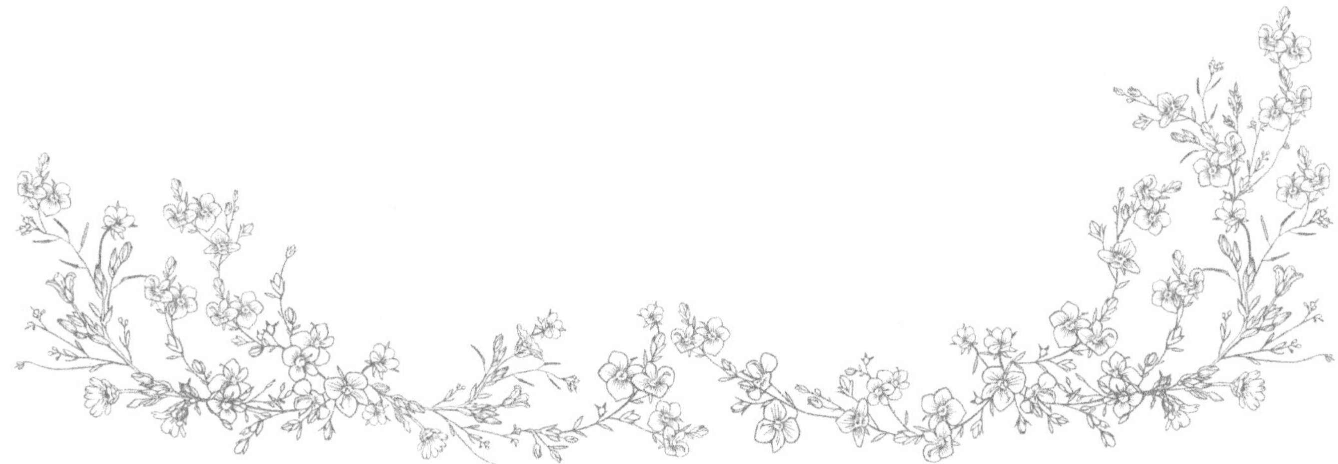

Garlic

Allium sativum (Liliaceae)

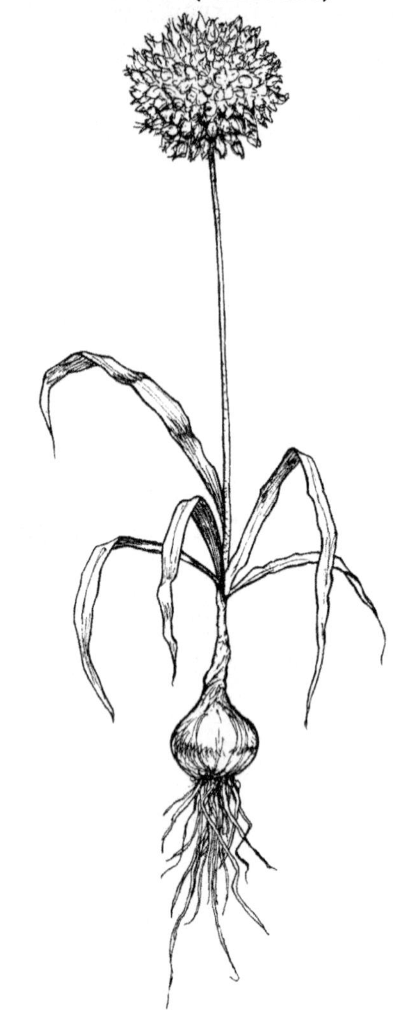

Any kitchen pantry cannot be complete without garlic. I always grab a couple of bulbs whenever I go to the farmers market. Garlic is a common ingredient added to everyday dishes. Its pungent odor and uniquely tangy taste contribute to a distinct flavor in any meal.

I also keep garlic in my apothecary because it is beneficial and versatile in herbalism. It can offer incredible health benefits like preventing heart problems, keeping your blood pressure in check, and lowering blood sugar and cholesterol *(Goncagul & Ayaz, 2010)*. The pungent odor and taste of raw garlic may not be tolerated well by some people, so take caution.

Description

We may all be familiar with garlic bulbs, but it is also essential to identify the plant itself. The long stalk of the plant sprouts from a flowering bulb, also called a head or knob. At the top of the stem, it is adorned with greenish-white or pink flowers. The leaves are long, flat, and grasslike, and the plant can grow as tall as 18–24 inches (45.72–60.96 centimeters).

History

I gained a greater appreciation for garlic when I viewed it from a historical perspective. Garlic had a significant role in ancient Egypt, Rome, China, and Greece. In Egypt, Greece, and Rome, it was given to soldiers and the working class as part of their everyday diet and was believed to increase stamina and strength. Ancient Chinese medicine used it to aid respiratory and digestive conditions, including diarrhea and worm infections *(Rivlin, 2001)*. This herb was even mentioned in the Bible as one of the things Jewish enslaved people missed once they fled Egypt.

Habitat & Cultivation

Although garlic is now widely cultivated worldwide, its original habitat was Central Asia. As most garlic flowers fade before they can produce seeds, it is recommended that you grow your garlic from the clove. To grow garlic in your herbal garden, separate a clove from a bulb and plant it, preferably in autumn or spring *(Catherine et al., 2021)*. If your plant thrives, you can harvest them by late summer.

Active Compounds: Scordinins; Selenium; Volatile oils

Herbal Actions: Anthelmintic; Antibiotics; Antidiabetic; Enhances sweating; Expectorant; Lowers blood pressure

Parts Used: Cloves

Main Use:

- Antibiotic for infectious illnesses
- Digestive infections and intestinal parasites management
- Can keep your blood thin, which helps prevent circulatory problems and minimizes the risk of stroke.

Self-care Use:

- Topically used for acne, boils, athlete's foot, or fungal infection
- Colds, flu, digestive infections, and urinary infection

⚠ Caution!

★ Can give a burning sensation to the skin or cause severe irritation.

★ Too much garlic intake can lead to heartburn, gas, bad breath, or diarrhea.

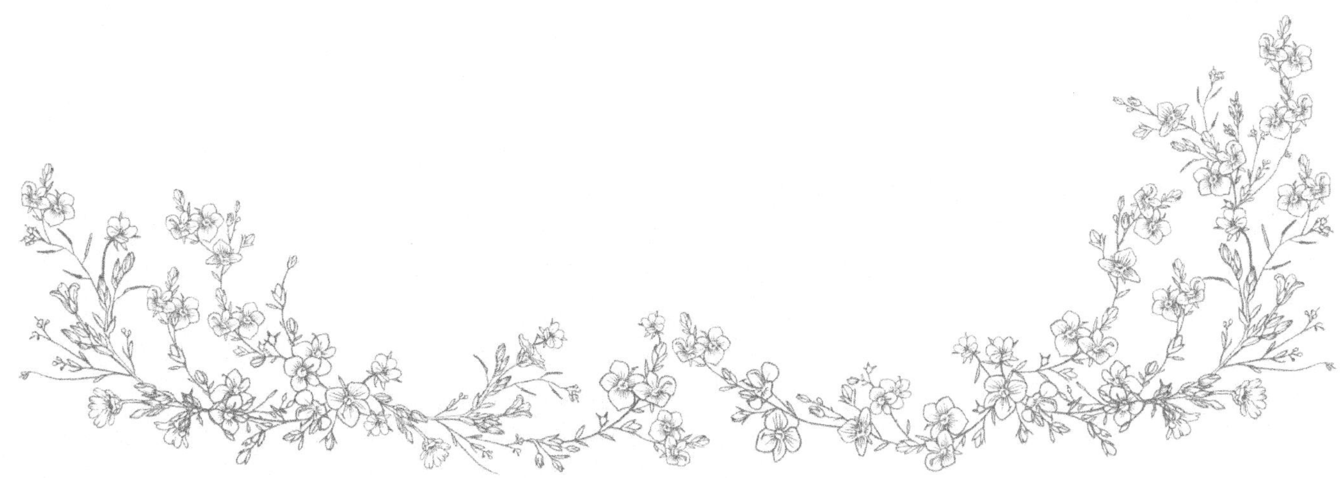

Ginkgo

Ginkgo biloba (Ginkgoaceae)

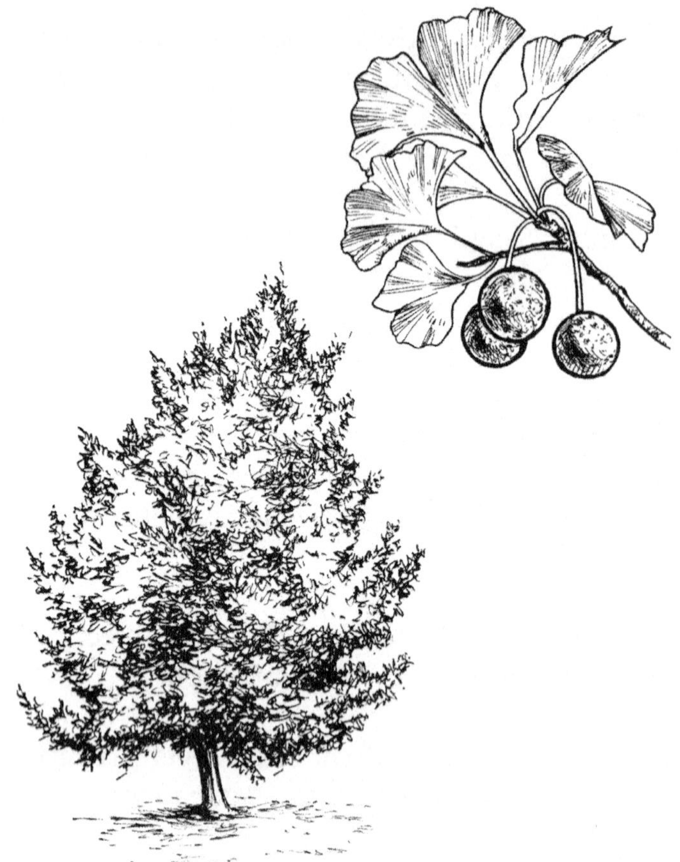

Ginkgo is a well-known herb with many health benefits and has been used in herbal remedies for a long time. Some conditions it may help with are cardiovascular problems, vertigo, breast tenderness, and other symptoms related to PMS *(Encyclopedia.com, 2018)*. If you want a tincture filled with powerful antioxidants for your heart health and circulation, try using ginkgo leaves.

Some studies have shown that its high antioxidants may help with cognitive issues like Alzheimer's and Dementia. However, researchers have much controversy about its effectiveness in slowing down changes in the brain.

Description

Gingko grows into a pyramidal-shaped tree and can reach up to 100 feet (30 meters) tall. The sparse branches are adorned with fan-shaped leaves that have a leathery feel. Its bark is corky textured and gets darker as the tree ages.

History

Ginkgo is one of the oldest tree species on earth. It is said that it even existed before the dinosaurs! It is the sole survivor of its species and has been called a "living fossil" *(Hill, 2018)*. Since it originated in Asia, the Chinese and Japanese have used ginkgo to help strengthen kidneys and bladders, improve digestion, and treat respiratory conditions.

Written records indicated its transplantation to the United States in 1784, but archaeological evidence shows some form of the species was there far before that time. You can still see one of the oldest ginkgo fossil forests on the banks of the Columbia River in Washington state.

Habitat & Cultivation

Ginkgo is cultivated in numerous areas of the world. This resilient tree can grow well in urban conditions and tolerate pollution and pests. If you want to produce a ginkgo tree at home, you can start from seed, but it will not be easy. Also, you will not be able to determine the sex of your tree for nearly 30 years. If you obtain a cutting, you will get a better result, and propagation from cuttings will allow you to pick the sex of your tree. The best time to take cuttings is during mid-summer. Make sure your plants have moist, well-draining soil, like a mixture of sand and perlite or peat moss.

Active Compounds: Bilobalides; Flavonoids; Ginkgolides

Herbal Actions: Anti-allergenic; Anti-asthmatic; Anti-inflammatory; Antispasmodic; Circulatory tonic

Parts Used: Seeds; Leaves (fresh or dried)

Main Use:

- Manage vaginal discharge and incontinence
- Extracts may help blood circulation in the brain
- Reduce the risk of stroke: strengthening nerve tissue and blood circulation

Self-care Use:

- Seeds can be processed to manage wheezing and phlegm.
- Leaves can relieve symptoms of asthma.
- It can be used in boosting memory, managing high blood pressure and arteriosclerosis.

⚠ **Caution!**

★ Be mindful of the dose taken since toxic reactions may occur.
★ May interact with medications like blood-thinners.
★ DO NOT eat fresh seeds; it may cause death. ☠
★ DO NOT take ginkgo if you have EVER had a seizure.

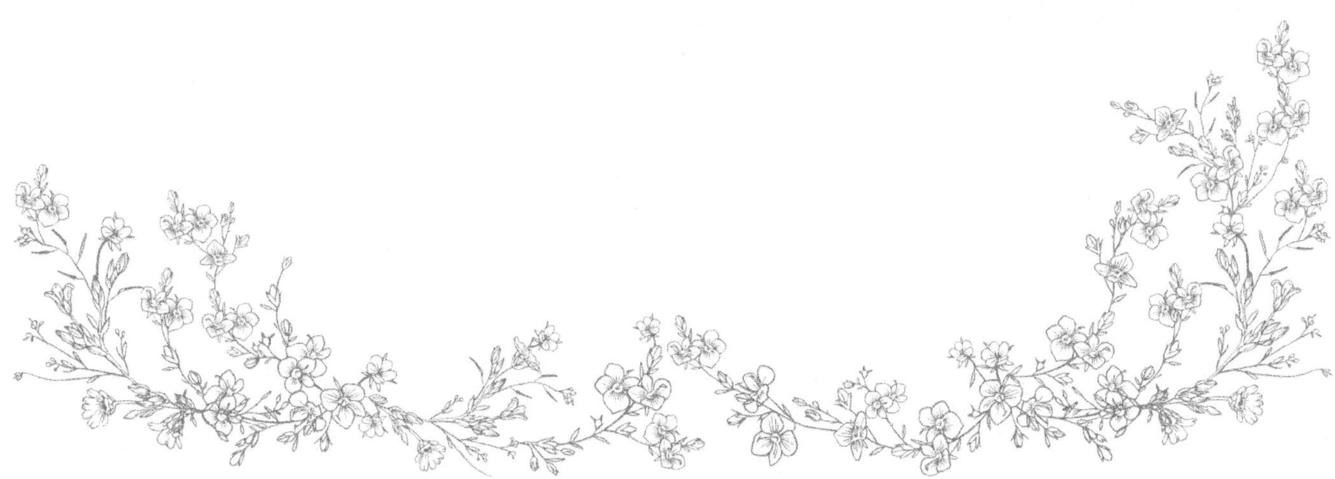

Goldenseal

Hydrastis canadensis (Ranunculaceae)

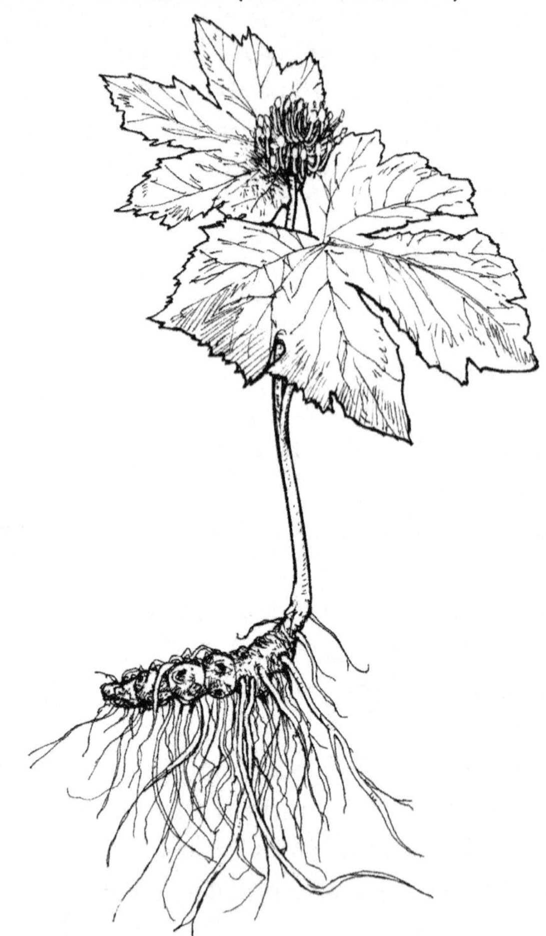

Goldenseal rhizomes are the part of this plant used most frequently for different herbal preparations. The extracted active compounds are antibacterial and may be helpful for digestive upset, such as constipation or diarrhea. Tea, capsules, or other extracts of goldenseal are used for infections and inflammation *(Petre, 2020)*. It is also an active ingredient in ear drops, eyewash, and allergy aids.

Description

Goldenseal is a small perennial and has a distinct yellow or golden-colored rhizome. This plant can grow 6–12 inches (less than 1 meter) tall with shiny, green-colored leaves. It has singular white flowers, which can be seen all over the plant.

History

Goldenseal has a rich history of being a powerful healing agent. The Cherokee Indians utilized its rhizomes to manage snakebites and cancer. In 1798, the first documentation of Native Americans using goldenseal for cancer was noted in *Essays Toward a Materia Medica of the United States (McCracken, n.d.)*. Other Native American Tribes used it for eye infections, mouth sores, liver trouble, digestive disorders, and even pneumonia. The early American settlers learned much about the many uses of this powerful herb from Native Americans.

Habitat & Cultivation

Goldenseal is native to North America and thrives in moist, mountainous regions. The popularity of this excellent plant has made it prone to overharvesting in the wild. Hence, it has become rare and, in 1991, was put on the endangered plant list.

If you choose to grow this herb in your garden, it is best planted in the shade. It needs rich loamy soil that is moist and has excellent drainage. It will need to be covered with mulch in the winter to help maintain the moisture levels. Rhizomes of goldenseal can be cultivated by dividing them every 3–5 years. You can also develop plants from seed, but it will take up to 2 years to grow harvestable rhizomes.

Active Compounds: Isoquinoline alkaloids; Resin; Volatile oil

Herbal Actions: Antibacterial; Anti-inflammatory; Bitter tonic

Parts Used: Rhizome (fresh or dried)

Main Use:

- Maintains healthy mucous membranes in the eyes, ears, nose, throat, and gastrointestinal tract.

Self-care Use:

- May help reduce excessive menstrual bleeding.
- Gargle decoctions for management of sore throat.
- Alleviates digestive problems and inflammation.

⚠ **Caution!**

★ Avoid taking in large doses.
★ DO NOT take if PREGNANT or breastfeeding
★ DO NOT give to children.
★ Avoid taking if you have hypertension

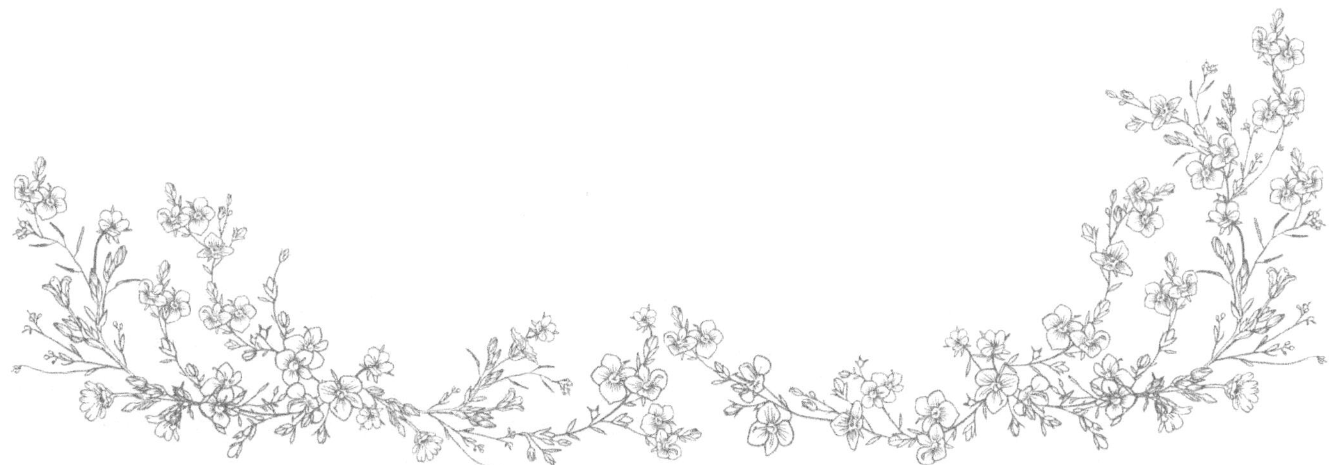

Hawthorn

Crataegus oxyacantha & C. monogyna (Rosaceae)

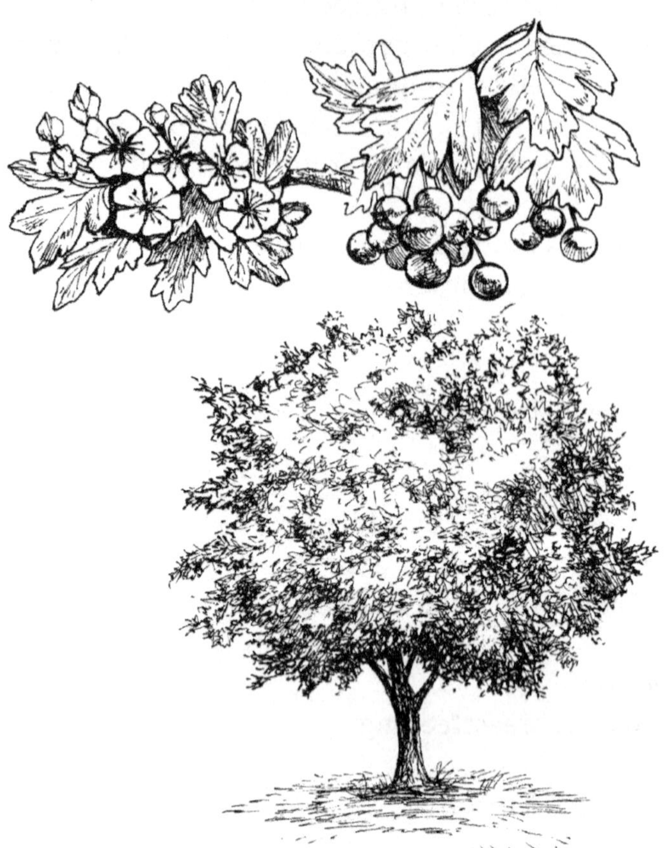

Hawthorn herbal extracts have proven to help manage heart problems in some cases. Although currently, there is not enough research to show that this herb can reduce mortality and sudden death of people suffering from chronic heart conditions. For this reason, it is imperative to consult your primary health physician before taking hawthorn. Those who suffer from congestive heart failure should never take this herb.

Another documented use of hawthorn is found in Chinese medicine, where it is prepared into jelly, jam, wine, or candies to help digestion *(Dahmer & Scott, 2015)*. Similarly, I like to sip hawthorn tea when I have a bit of indigestion.

Description

Hawthorn is a spiny plant with scaly bark that can grow up to 5 feet (about 1.5 meters) tall. It is a deciduous plant with toothed or lobed simple leaves that grow from thorny branches. In the spring, pink, white, or red flowers blossom in small clusters, followed by small berries called "haws" in autumn. These berries can range from blue or black to red or orange.

History

Physicians praised hawthorn as far back as the 1st century when Dioscorides wrote of its power to aid heart problems. Throughout the centuries, research on the validity of early historical assertions continued to develop *(Freed, 2017)*. By the early 19th century, the claims were concluded, finding hawthorn was valuable for regulating blood pressure, increasing blood flow to the heart, increasing the strength of heart contractions, and decreasing blood lipids.

Habitat & Cultivation

Hawthorn is native to most of Europe, West Asia, and North Africa but can be cultivated worldwide in a suitable climate. It typically grows in temperate climates, and one can see it growing wild along roadsides or fields.

This plant is generally not very picky with how it develops. Make sure you plant your hawthorn in rich, well-draining soil with plenty of space and sun to ensure it will thrive. You can cultivate it from seeds but expect it to take around 18 months for them to germinate. The long waiting time is lessened by acquiring tree cuttings instead. Take your cuttings in June or July and root them before planting.

Active Compounds: Polyphenols; Proanthocyanins; Bioflavonoids; Triterpenoids; Coumarine; Amines

Herbal Actions: Circulatory tonic; Antioxidant; Lowers blood pressure; Diuretic

Parts Used: Flowers; Berries; Leaves

Main Use:

- Helps manage kidney and bladder stones.
- Helps manage heart issues: coronary heart disease and angina.

Self-care Use:

- Taking a tea, tincture, or decoction can help normalize blood pressure.
- Combining hawthorn with gingko biloba may help boost memory retention.

⚠ **Caution!**

★ It may interact with some medications for the heart, blood pressure, and cholesterol.

★ DO NOT take if you have congestive heart failure

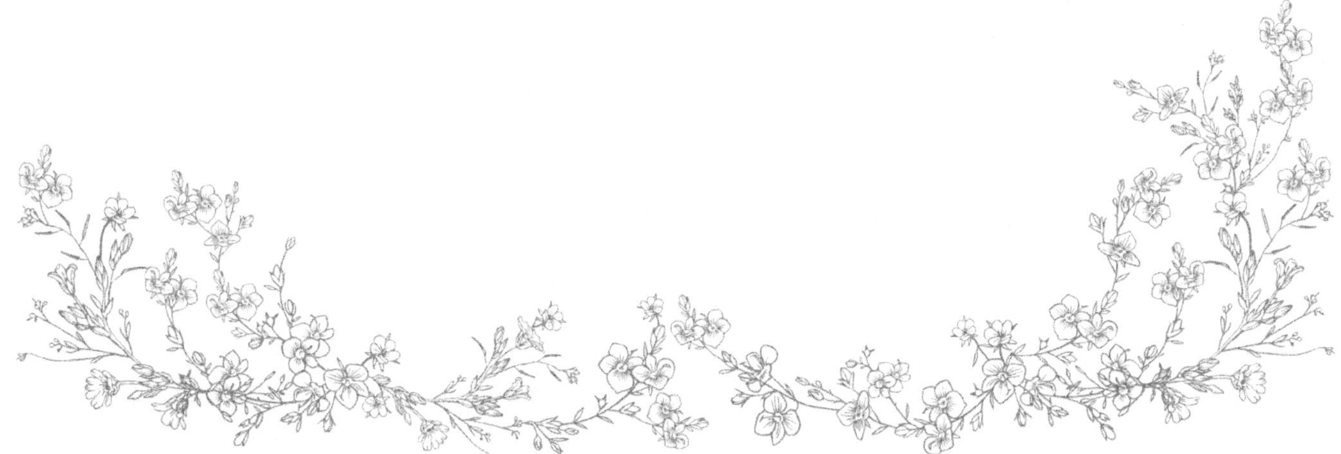

Licorice

Glycyrrhiza glabra (Fabaceae)

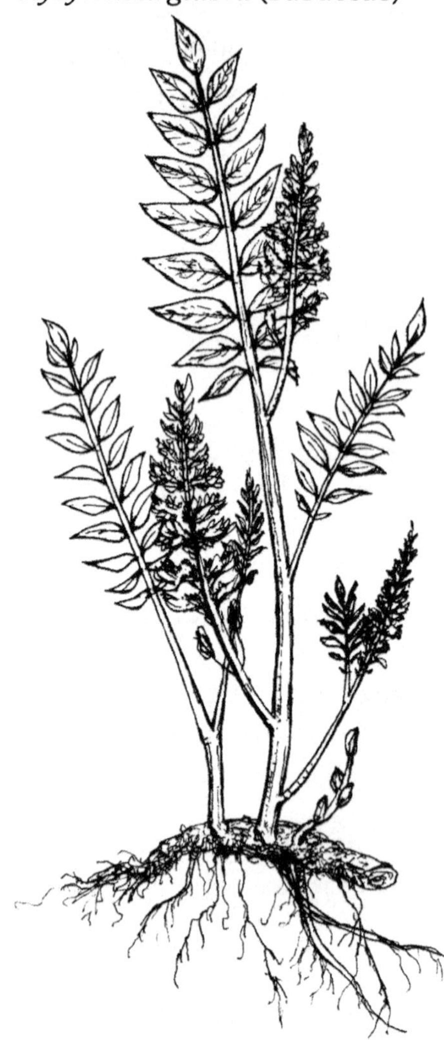

If you are like me, who has a sweet tooth, licorice can be a go-to herbal solution for your need for sweets. Licorice, especially its roots, is surprisingly sweet because of its glycyrrhizic acid content. This chemical compound is noted to be a lot sweeter than table sugar. Aside from this, its anti-inflammatory capabilities also make it helpful for gastritis, arthritis, and canker sores.

Description

Licorice is a mounding plant that grows 1.5–3 feet (about 46–91.4 centimeters) tall. It has smooth, teardrop-shaped leaves that arrange themselves opposite each other and can have anywhere from 7–12 leaflets along one stem. These leaves are typically bright green, and the plant will produce cream-colored flower heads if left to blossom. The part of the plant most often used is the roots, which are small rhizomes harvested at about 3 feet (1 meter) long.

History

Because of the sweet taste of licorice root, it was used as a sweet drink for Egyptian pharaohs in Ancient Egypt. In a more therapeutic aspect, it was utilized by the Ancient Greeks, Chinese, and Middle Easterners to alleviate inflammation and help problems in the stomach and upper respiratory systems. These applications are mostly how modern society uses licorice today.

Habitat & Cultivation

This plant is native to West Asia and Southern Europe. Licorice grows flowers that look like peas; however, the most valuable herbal benefits are extracted from their roots. Propagating licorice is also quite simple – its roots can be divided and planted. You can dig out the roots of 3–4-year-old licorice during late autumn to maximize the active compounds.

Active Compounds: Isoflavones; Phytosterols; Polysaccharides; Triterpene saponins

Herbal Actions: Anti-inflammatory; Demulcent; Expectorant; Mild laxative

Parts Used: Root (fresh or dried)

Main Use:

- Traditionally used for asthma, chest pains, and canker sores.
- Soothes the digestive tract.
- Soothes inflammation in the eyes or joints.

Self-care Use:

- Can be consumed to aid constipation, coughs, or bronchitis.
- Can alleviate the loss of appetite.

⚠ **Caution!**

- ★ Some consequences of taking large doses include increased blood pressure.
- ★ Seek professional advice if you plan to take while PREGNANT

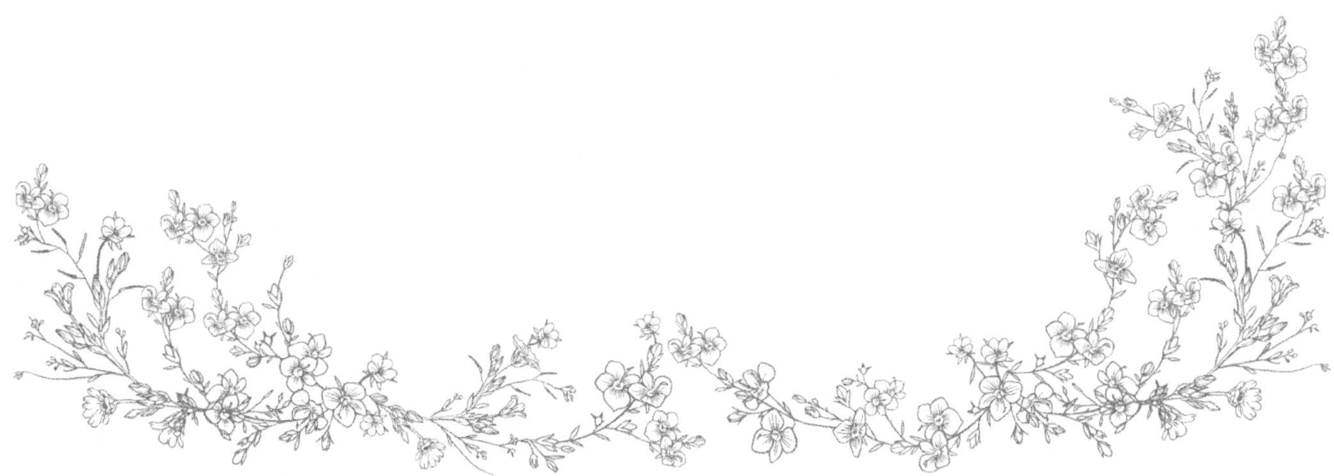

Milk Thistle

Silybum marianum (Asteraceae)

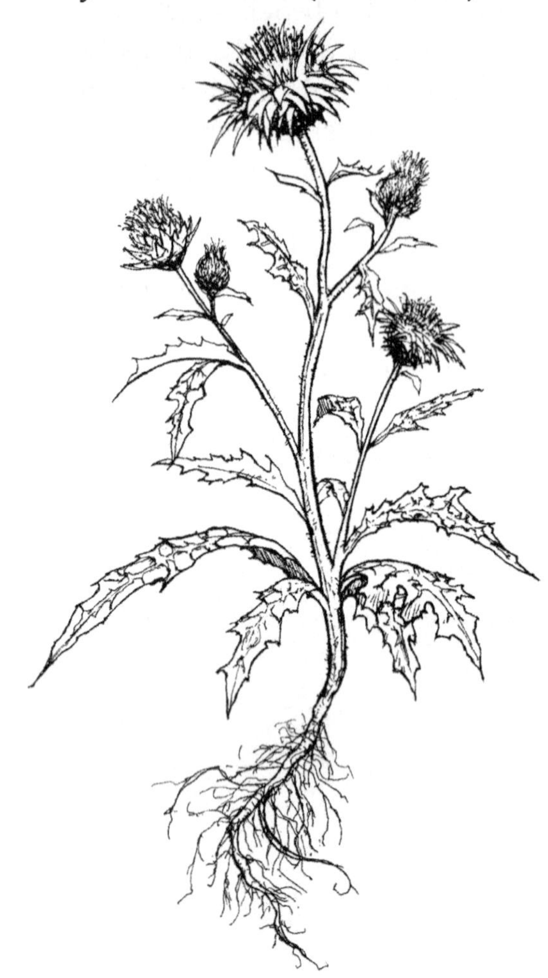

Do not be intimidated by the spiny appearance of milk thistle; it provides us with many health benefits! It can promote liver and skin health, reduce cholesterol and insulin resistance, and help bones stay healthy *(Burgess, 2017)*. The pretty flowers of milk thistle and its seeds hold most of the active ingredients that give these benefits.

Description

Milk thistle comes from the same plant family as daisies and can grow up to 6.5 feet (2 meters) tall. It has brightly colored magenta and purple flowerheads. The base of the flowerheads has very thick and spiny bracts. Sharp spines also erupt from the leaves and stems.

History

Milk thistle has been appreciated for its medicinal properties for nearly 2000 years. As far back as the 1st century, written recordings of its use for liver protection were noted. It also became a go-to plant for gallbladder and spleen ailments in early Europe and was frequently used throughout the Middle Ages *(Encyclopedia.com, 2018)*. These are remarkable findings because modern studies have backed up these claims.

Habitat & Cultivation

Milk thistle grows in Mediterranean regions and Europe. Besides growing wild, this herb can be an ornamental plant for your herbal garden. Although, they have been given a bad reputation as a weed because they tend to reseed fast if not harvested promptly after flowering. Using their flowerheads will be optimum during early summer, while seeds are harvested during late summer when the flower heads begin to dry and turn brown.

Active Compounds: Bitter principles; Flavonolignans; Polyacetylenes

Herbal Actions: Anti-allergenic; Anti-cancer; Chemoprotective; Hepatoprotective

Parts Used: Seeds and flowerheads

Main Use:

- Liver problems: jaundice and hepatitis

Self-care Use

- Tinctures can help hay fever.
- Tablets for liver disorders.
- Flowerheads can be eaten like fresh vegetables.
- May aid breastmilk production and melancholia.

⚠ **Caution!**

★ Can cause allergic reactions.

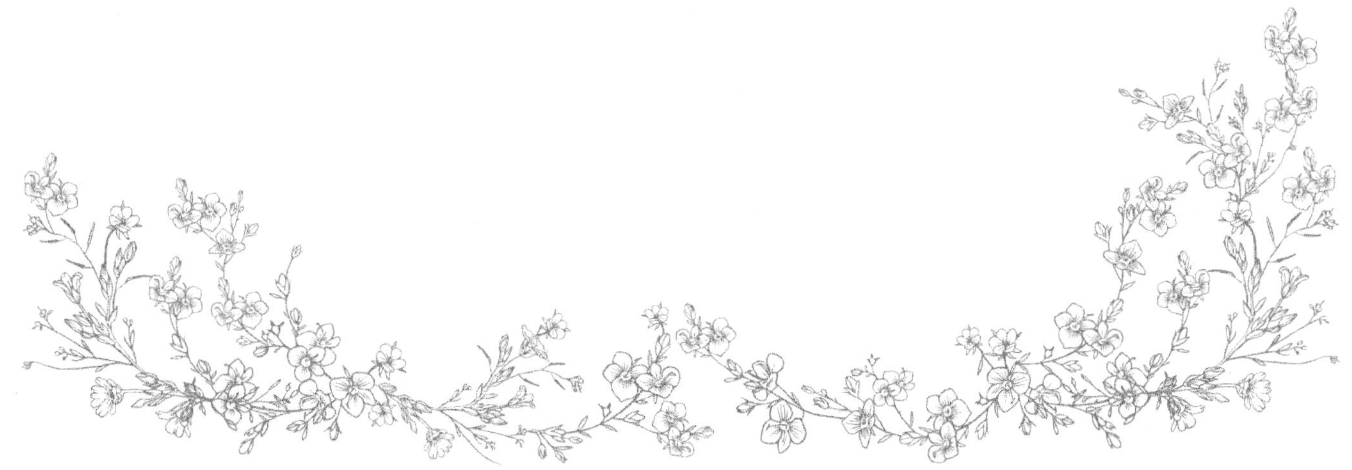

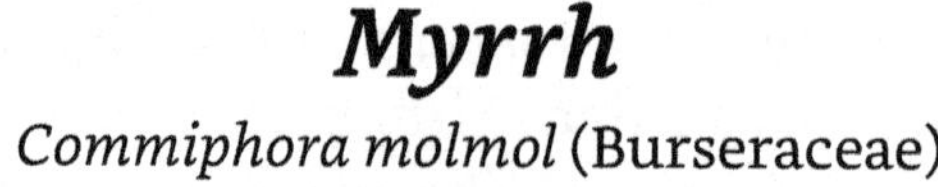

Myrrh

Commiphora molmol (Burseraceae)

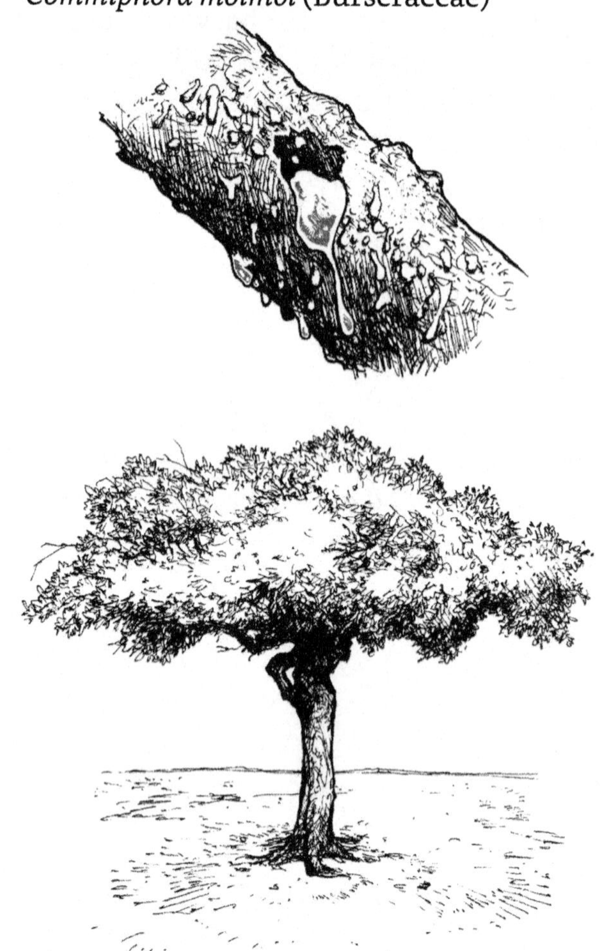

Myrrh is not a plant but a thick and yellow-colored resin of the *Commiphora molmol* tree. This resin is very aromatic and widely used in perfumes and incense. Of course, it also has some medicinal uses, such as killing bacteria, pain relief, and the reduction of swelling. It can undergo steam distillation to extract its essential oils.

Description

Commiphora molmol can grow into a massive 16-foot (5 meters) tall tree with a light-gray-colored trunk. It has twisted branches with leaves that have rough and sharp edges. These solitary trees thrive among rocks and sand in hot desert regions.

History

The fragrance of myrrh resin made it a well-used ingredient in perfumes and holy ointments. Ancient Chinese medicine used it to treat wounds, relieve swelling, and manage menstrual cramps *(Encylopedia.com, 2018).* These applications are very close to how we utilize this plant in the modern era.

A more familiar historical note of myrrh is its mention in the New Testament. Myrrh, along with gold and frankincense, was part of the three gifts offered by the magi to Christ on the day of his birth.

Habitat & Cultivation

Commiphora molmol is native to Northeast Africa and other hot climates like Saudi Arabia, Iran, and India. This tree prefers to grow in well-draining, sandy soil with plenty of sunlight. If you decide to grow one at home, you will only need to water them once every other week for about 5-10 minutes. You can cultivate from seed, but propagating this tree from cuttings is easier.

Active Compounds: Gum – acidic polysaccharides; Resin; Volatile oils

Herbal Actions: Anti-inflammatory; Antiparasitic; Antiseptic; Anti-ulcer; Astringent; Wound healer

Parts Used: Gum resin

Main Use:

- Astringent: sore throat, canker sores, and gingivitis.
- Considered for its aphrodisiac capabilities.

Self-care Use:

- Topically applied on acne, boils, oral ulcers, and oral thrush.

⚠ **Caution!**

- ★ Watch your dose! A very large intake may be harmful.

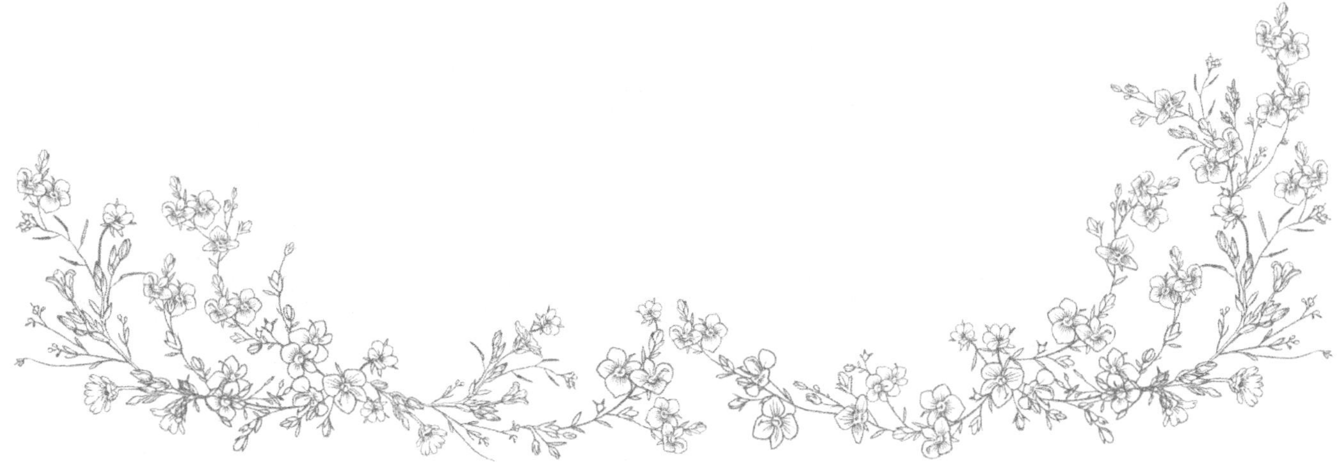

Nettle

Urtica dioica (Urticaceae)

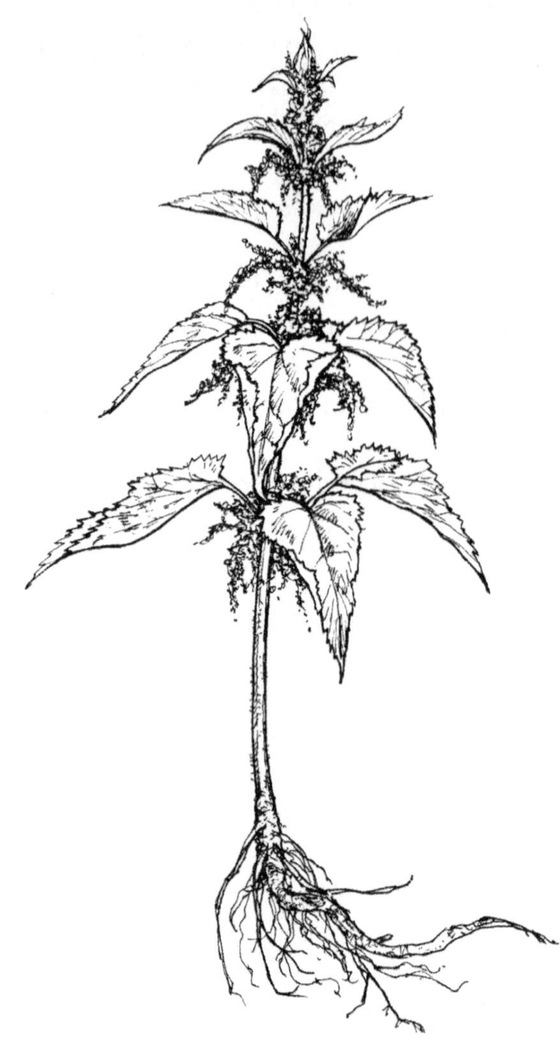

Every part of the nettle plant is usable! Nettle leaves hold the majority of active ingredients that provide health benefits. Seasonal allergies can be a big bummer, but not when I have my nettle tea and tincture to save the day. My sneezing fits, runny nose, and itchy eyes go away completely when I take nettle regularly during allergy season.

Description

Nettel can grow to around 6.5 feet (2 meters) tall and is usually a light green to tan color. It has toothed leaves that grow on opposite sides of its thinly tapered stems. These leaves and stems have a rough appearance and are covered in stinging hair, which is why this plant is commonly called "stinging nettle."

History

Records of nettle have been noted as far back as the Bronze Age. Later, during the reign of Julius Caesar, military troops used this herb to stay alert during the night *(Gaia Herb Farm, 2021).* Dioscorides also described the many uses of nettle during the 1st century, including its potential for managing wounds and stimulating menstruation.

Habitat & Cultivation

Stinging nettle is common in Europe, North Africa, and North America. Currently, it is prevalent worldwide, especially in Asian regions. Nettle shoots and leaves are harvested during summer and may be used as a dish ingredient and in herbal remedy preparations.

Active Compounds: Amines; Flavonoids; Glucoquinone; Minerals; Phenols; Plant sterols

Herbal Actions: Anti-allergenic; Anti-inflammatory; Astringent; Diuretic; Prevent hemorrhaging; Tonic

Parts Used: All parts

Main Use:

- Combined with other anti-inflammatory products to alleviate osteoarthritis symptoms.
- May have a positive effect on enlarged prostate and urinary tract issues.

Self-care Use:

- Ointment: topically applied to areas with eczema
- Has anti-allergenic properties: hay fever, asthma, and bites and stings.
- Used to slow or stop bleeding

⚠ **Caution!**

- ★ Stingy stems and leaves may cause irritation to the skin

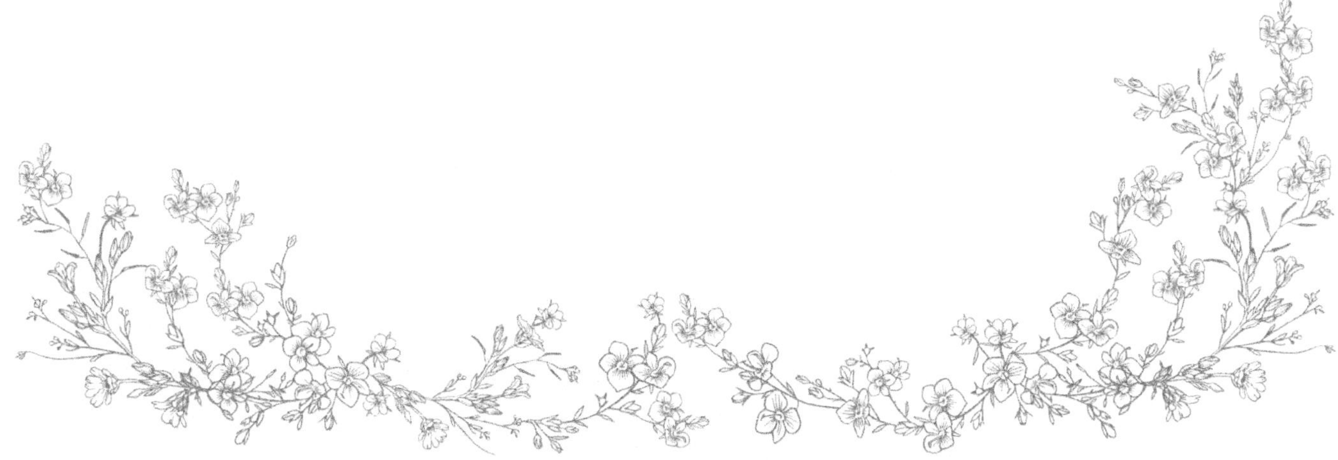

Peppermint

Minta x piperita (Lamiaceae)

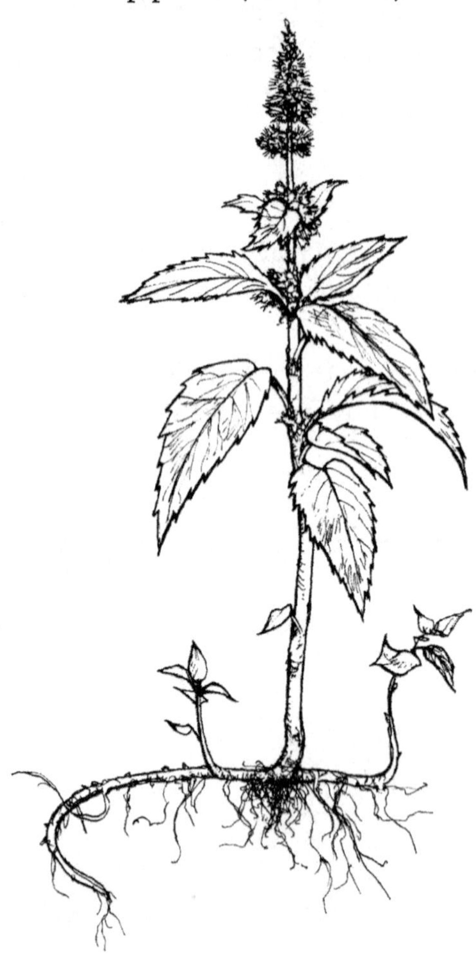

I genuinely adore the extracted essential oils from peppermint. It has a calming scent that puts me in a relaxed mood, especially after a tiring day. It also benefits the digestive tract, which is great because I like to eat foods that do not always agree with my stomach. Also, peppermint tea is caffeine-free, so I know I can have it right before bed, and it will not keep me up all night.

Description

Peppermint is a plant with a strong minty aroma and typically grows to around 3 feet (1 meter) tall. Common to all plants in the mint family, peppermint has distinct square stems with dark green leaves. When these plants grow, they aggressively dominate due to the growth pattern of their underground stems.

History

Different species of mint have been used throughout the centuries and are noted as one of the oldest cultivated medicinal plants. Japanese records show that it has been in use for nearly 2000 years! From ancient Japan and Egypt to Rome and Greece, this herb was used for numerous ailments. A few benefits mentioned in these ancient cultures were its ability to help with stomach or abdominal pain and assist with gall bladder ailments.

Habitat & Cultivation

This aromatic herb is native to Europe and Asia, but because of its popularity, it is now grown worldwide. If you cultivate peppermint at home, it is recommended to plant it in a container, so it does not take over your garden. The best time to harvest the plant for oil extraction is springtime.

Active Compounds: Flavonoids; Phenolic acids; Triterpenes; Volatile oils

Herbal Actions: Analgesic; Antimicrobial; Antispasmodic; Carminative; Perspirant

Parts Used: Aerial parts (fresh or dried)

Main Use:

- Used for relaxing gut muscles to reduce cramping, gas, and nausea.
- Antimicrobial: may aid in respiratory infections.

Self-care Use:

- Topically applied to the skin for pain alleviation.
- Diluted essential oil applied to the temples to ease headaches.

⚠ **Caution!**

★ Not recommended for children below five years of age.

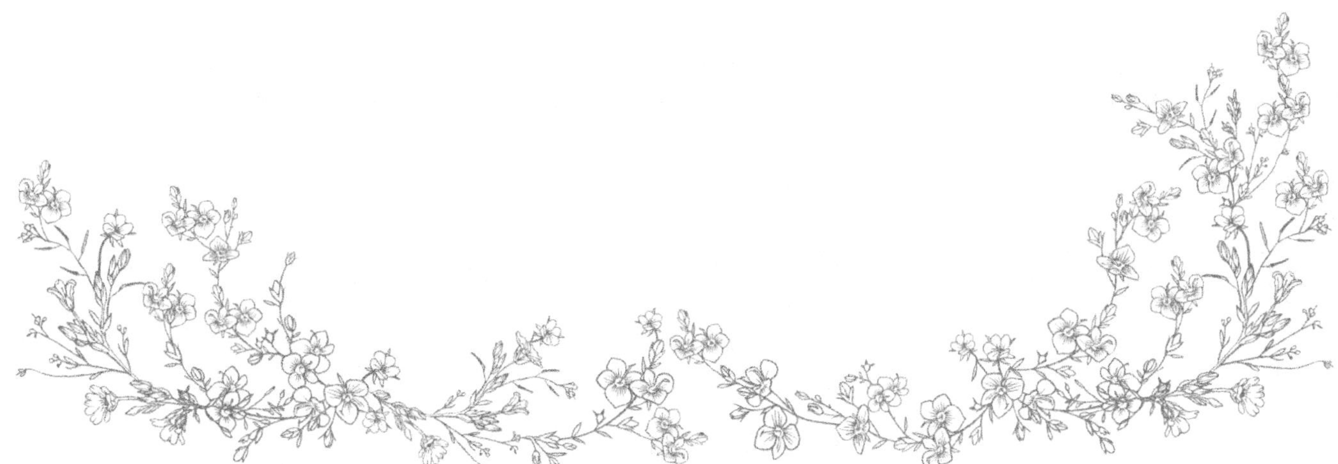

Quinoa

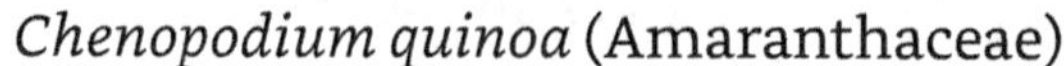
Chenopodium quinoa (Amaranthaceae)

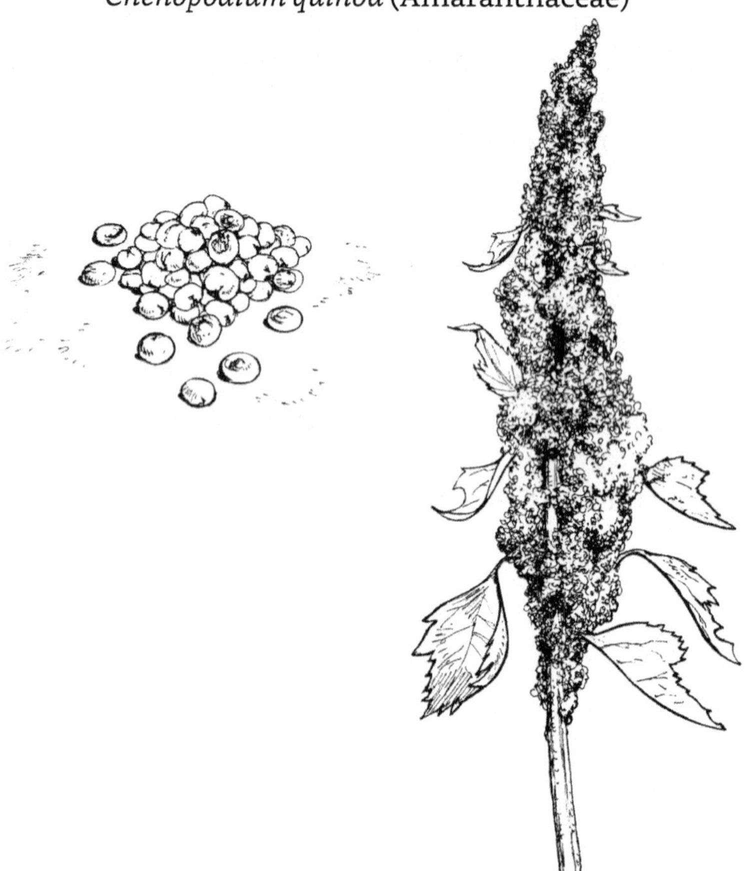

Quinoa is a flowering plant known for its edible seeds, rich in nutrients and dietary fibers. This pseudo-cereal is filled with protein and essential amino acids while remaining gluten-free *(Gunnars, 2018).* I switched rice out for quinoa a few years ago and have noticed a significant difference in my energy levels. Rice is good, but quinoa is much better and better for your health!

Description

Quinoa can grow up to 6.5 feet (2 meters) tall and has powdery or hairy lobed leaves placed alternatively along the stem. The woody center stem can be branched or unbranched and is green, red, or purple, depending on the variety. Seeds from quinoa plants, when cooked, look very similar to millets.

History

During the early times, quinoa was primarily used as food for livestock. Eventually, people started consuming it for its many different dietary benefits, including proteins, fibers, and minerals. For the Inca Empire, quinoa was called the “mother of all grains” because it was believed to be sacred *(Gunnars, 2018).* Eventually, quinoa reached the status of being a superfood after it became trendy in South America.

Habitat & Cultivation

Quinoa originated in South America, but because of its popularity, it is now cultivated in more than 70 countries globally. This plant grows well in areas with well-distributed rainfall during its early growth stages. Minimal to no rain is optimal as the seed matures and reaches the harvesting stage.

Active Compounds: Flavonoids; Kaempferol; Quercetin

Herbal Actions: Anti-cancer; Anti-inflammatory; Antioxidants; Antiviral

Parts Used: Seeds and leaves

Main Use:

- Best for gluten intolerant individuals.

Self-care Use:

- Antioxidants and amino acids: daily snack
- Aid in blood sugar control in individuals with low glycemic index

⚠ **Caution!**

★ Can cause allergic reactions to individuals sensitive to other grains like wheat, rice, or buckwheat.

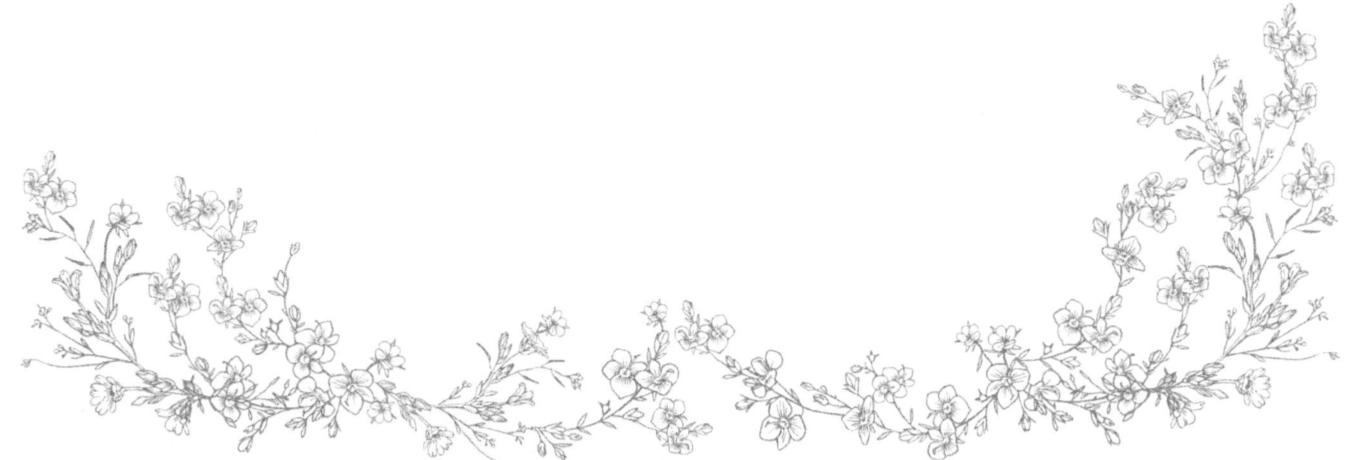

Sage

Salvia officinalis (Lamiaceae)

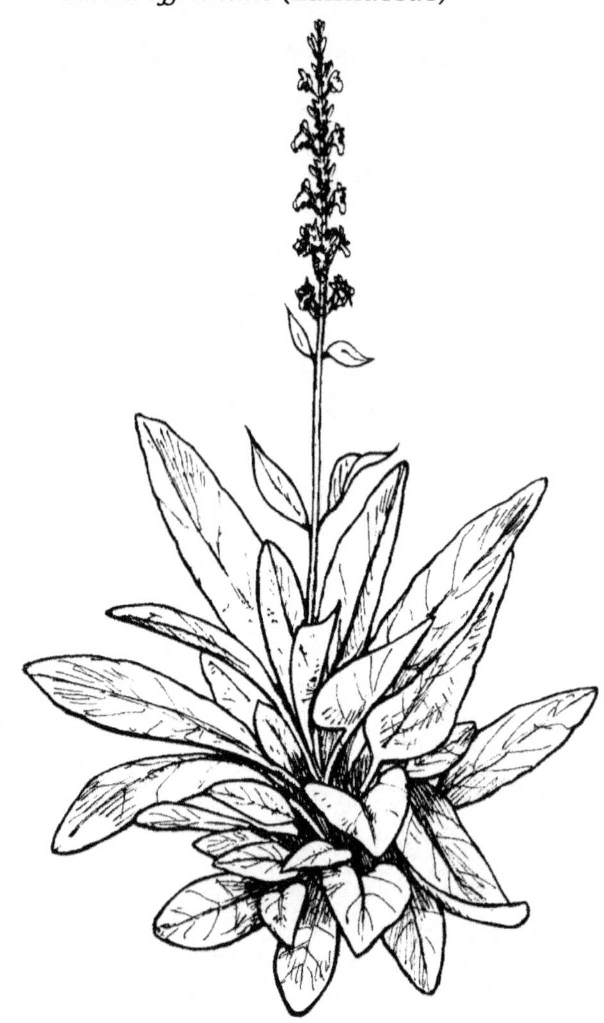

Sage is another one of my all-time favorite herbs, as there are over 700 species of *Salvia* plants. It belongs to the mint family and has a sweet aroma and earthy flavor, making it a popular cooking herb. Aside from this, the leaves hold promising health benefits, including antiseptic and astringent potential.

Description

Salvia officinalis plants have square stems and ovate leaves, ranging in color between gray, green, and even purple. It usually grows to about 2 feet (0.61 meters) tall. Sage also has flowers that can have a variety of colors —red, pink, purple, or white. These particularly appeal to pollinators such as hummingbirds, bees, and butterflies.

History

Salvia, translated from Latin, means "to heal." In ancient times people thought that because sage had such a capacity to heal, a man with it in his home was not in danger of dying from any illness. The Ebers Papyrus (1500 BC) noted its ability to alleviate itching, while during Hippocrates' time, it was praised for its potential to aid with menstruation. Famous pharmacologists, such as Dioscorides and Galen, also noted the many uses of sage during the 1st century *(Vogel, 2021)*. The use of sage spanned the ages and is still prevalent today.

Habitat & Cultivation

The shores of the northern Mediterranean are the original home of common sage, but because of its popularity, it is now cultivated worldwide. If you want to grow it at home, the best way to grow it is from a cutting. Your plants will need plenty of sunlight and sandy, loamy soil that is not too wet. Sage is drought resistant and does not like to be overwatered! Harvest your leaves in summer for optimum benefits.

Active Compounds: Diterpenes; Essential oils; Phenolic compounds; Tannins; Triterpenes

Herbal Actions: Antiseptic; Astringent; Estrogenic

Parts Used: Leaves (dried or fresh)

Main Use:

- May enhance memory retention due to its nerve tonic capacity.
- Can promote better digestion.

Self-care Use:

- Sage infusions can be used as a gargle to aid sore throats.
- Fresh leaves can be rubbed on stings and bug bites.

⚠ **Caution!**

★ Not recommended for pregnant and breastfeeding women or epileptic individuals.

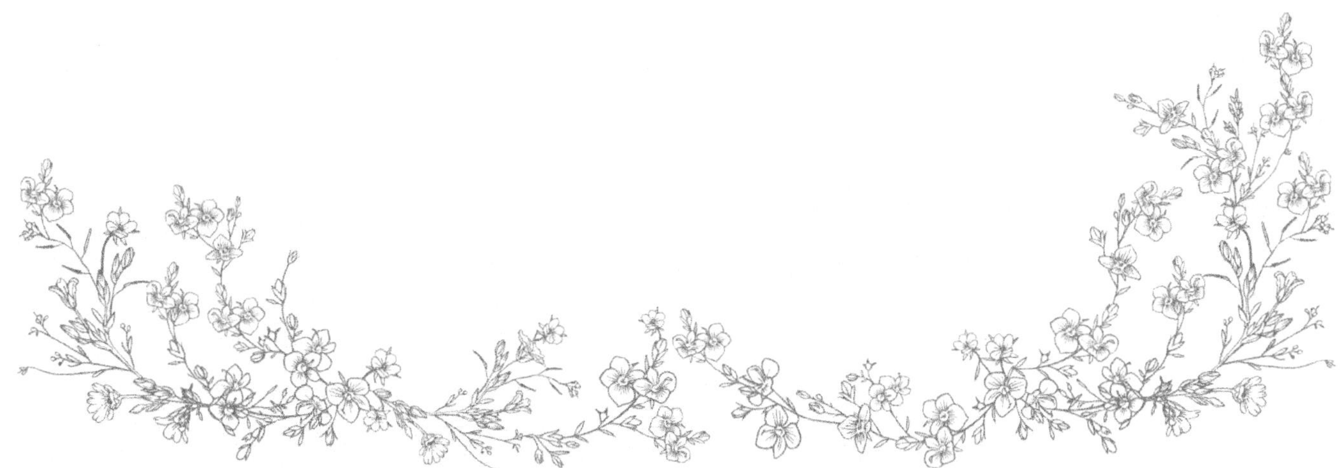

St. John's Wort

Hypericum perforatum (Hypericaceae)

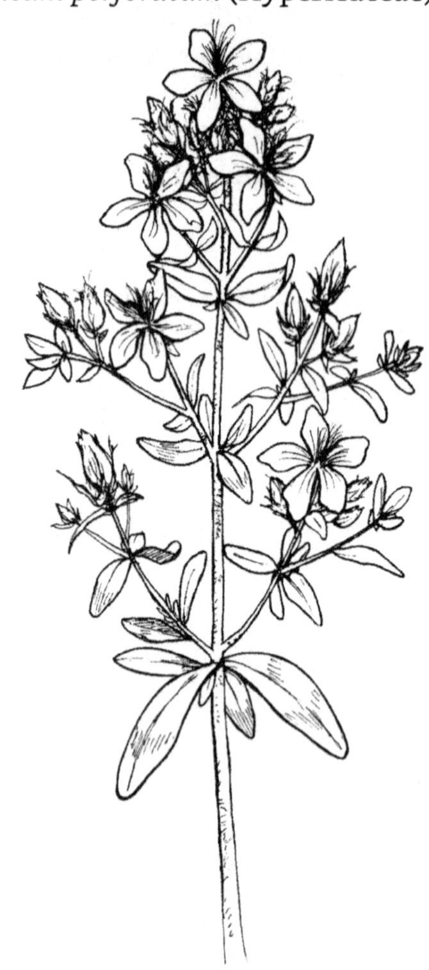

St. John's wort is a plant long used for depression, anxiety, and loss of motivation and appetite. Other applications include behavioral aids for obsessive-compulsive disorder and attention deficit hyperactivity disorder (ADHD). Although, these benefits are still currently undergoing research to probe deeper into what this herb does to help us.

Description

This plant is a low-lying herb that can grow up to 6 feet (1.83 meters) tall with bright yellow flower clusters. These flowers have five petals and small black dots scattered over the margins of each petal. It also has small, elliptical leaves which can be used for different herbal formulas. Interestingly, this herb turns bright red when infused with any oil!

History

St. John's wort gets its name from John the Baptist because it tends to be in full bloom around his birthday on June 24th *(Mount Sinai, 2021)*. This plant was used for powerful protection from lousy health and evil spirits in Medieval Europe. Fast forward to the 19th century, this herb is now believed to be practical for "all down-heartedness" – the modern application of the herb to alleviate depression and anxiety.

Habitat & Cultivation

This plant is considered native to Europe, the United States, and parts of Asia and Africa. St. John's Wort is known to thrive well in well-drained soil and prefers full sunlight. The main cultivation methods are from its seeds or root division. After successfully growing yours, you may harvest its flowering tops by summer.

Active Compounds: Flavonoids; Phloroglucinols; Polycyclic diones

Herbal Actions: Antidepressant; Anti-inflammatory; Antiviral

Parts Used: Flowers

Main Use:

- Neuroprotective for managing depressed mood and tiredness.
- Can promote healing in minor burns and as an adjunct to after-surgery wounds.

Self-care Use:

- Herb tinctures may aid depression, anxiety, and tension.
- Creams topically applied on areas of cramps, muscle aches, or neuralgia.

⚠ **Caution!**

★ Topical application may make skin more sensitive to sunlight.

★ DO NOT use if you are taking antidepressant medications

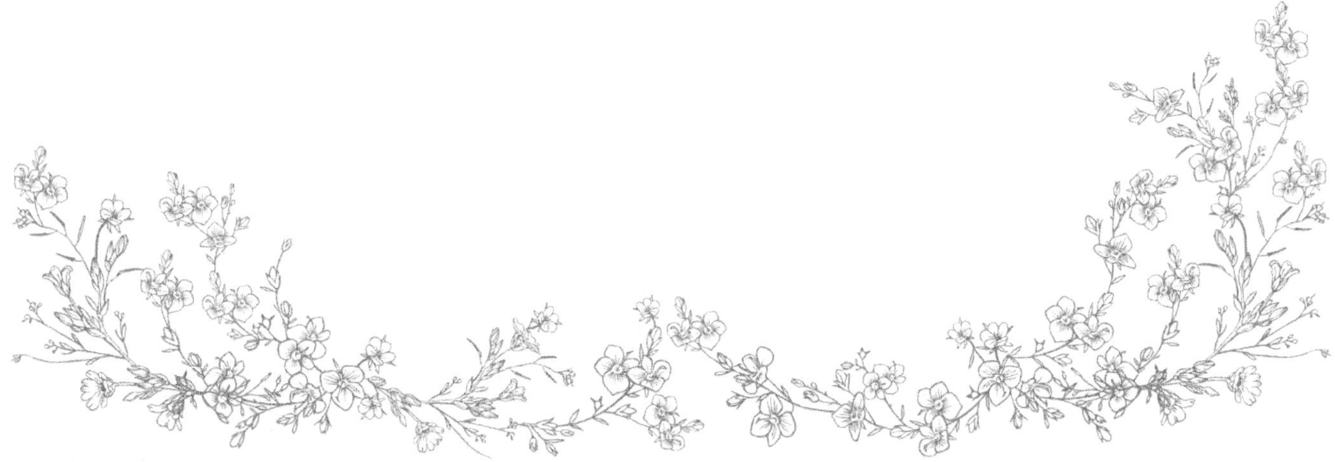

Yarrow

Achillea millefolium (Asteraceae)

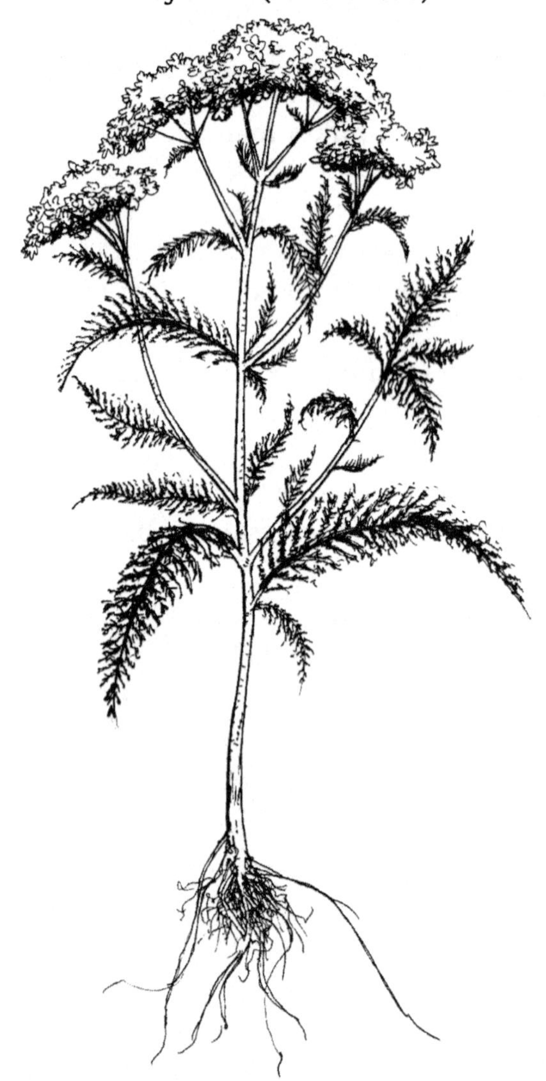

Navajo nations believe that yarrow is "life medicine" and use it for various ailments, like toothache and earache. Yarrow flowers contain volatile oils used in preparations like teas or essential oils. It has been noted to help with conditions such as wound healing, eczema, stomach aches, and irritable bowel syndrome (IBS). I find drinking yarrow tea soothes tummy pain and bloating while having a calming aroma.

Description

Achillea, the genus of yarrow, has 140 species! Common yarrow is a hardy perennial that grows up to 3 feet (1 meter) tall with delicate, aromatic, feathery-cut leaves. The dome-shaped clustered flowers can be seen in shades of yellow, pink, gold, and red, but most notably white.

History

This herb has numerous names, nosebleed, staunch weed, Achillea, and devil's nettle *(Dellwo, 2021)*. The multiple representations of yarrow are not surprising, knowing that different eras have employed this plant for its herbal properties. Native Americans have been utilizing this herb for centuries to aid in the healing of wounds. Furthermore, Greek mythology noted that Achilles used yarrow to help the injuries of his soldiers *(Bantillan, 2019)*. Hence, the name *Achillea*!

Habitat & Cultivation

It is thought that common yarrow is primarily native to Eurasia, but varieties are found worldwide. If you plan to plant this herb at home, be warned that it can be invasive because of its rhizomes' ability to spread fast. You might consider using a container unless you are okay with eventually having multiple yarrow plants. This plant is not too picky about its soil but prefers average to poor soil with a small amount of compost. Plant in full sunlight and harvest its aerial parts during summer.

Active Compounds: Alkaloids; Flavonoids; Sesquiterpene lactones; Tannins; Triterpenes; Volatile oils

Herbal Actions: Anti-inflammatory; Antispasmodic; Astringent

Parts Used: Aerial parts (fresh or dried)

Main Use:

- Promotes menstruation
- Stops internal bleeding

Self-care Use:

- Can clean wounds
- Can help manage fevers, colds, and flu
- Digestive infections

⚠ **Caution!**

★ Yarrows are generally safe, but it may cause skin irritation to sensitive individuals upon topical use.

★ Allergy to other Asteraceae plants may mean that you can also be allergic to yarrows.

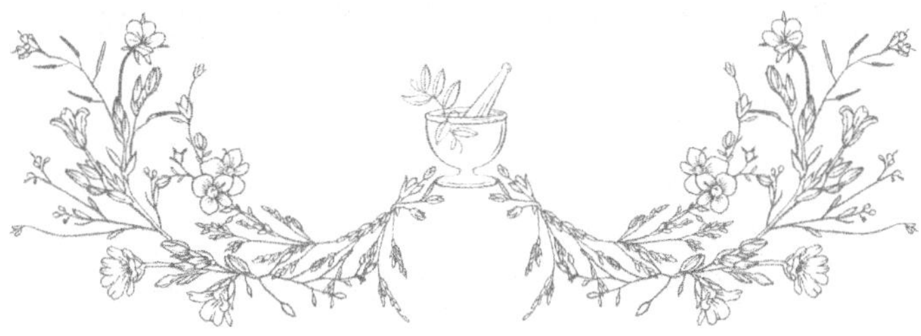

Herbs do not necessarily have to be rare or expensive. While some of the most widely beneficial herbs can be found in markets and grocery stores, wouldn't it be fun to learn how to grow, harvest, and store your own at home? Now that you are equipped with vital information about their various actions and uses, you are ready to start growing a simple herbal garden.

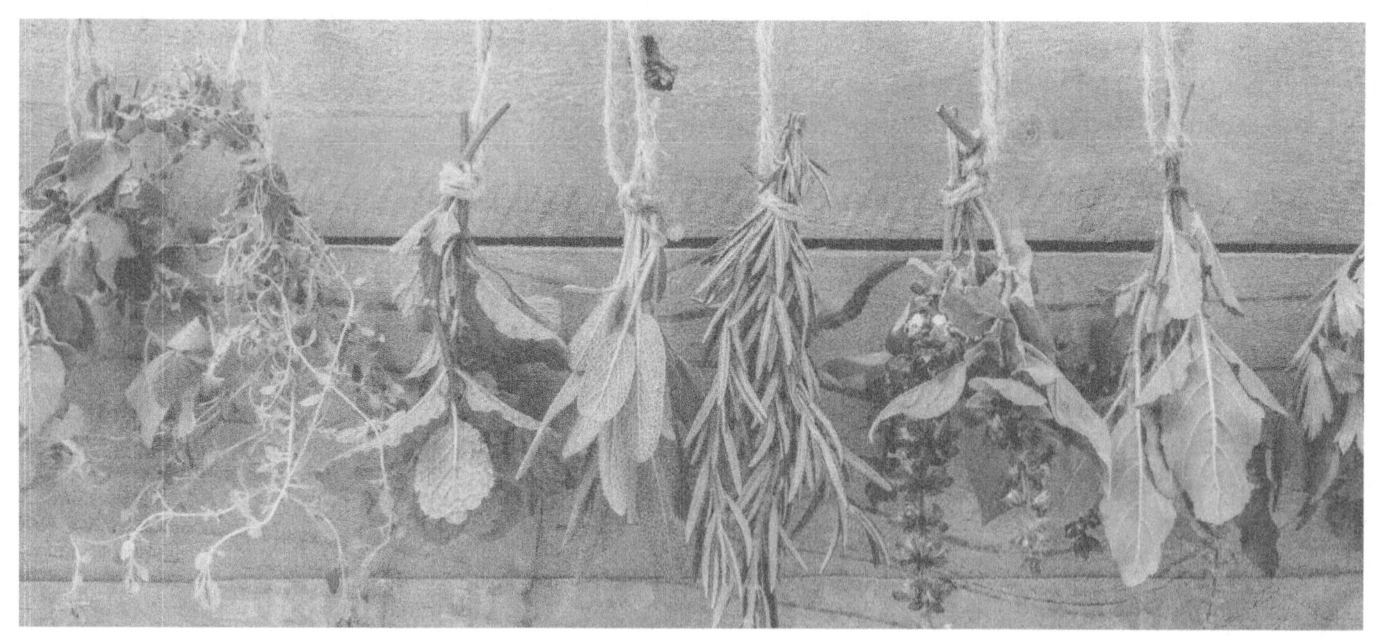

Chapter 7

How to Grow, Harvest & Store

After looking into the fantastic herbs in our previous chapters, you can cultivate each to prepare medicinal concoctions or added to your daily diet for overall wellness. When considering an herbal garden, ask yourself these simple questions: What types of herbs do you want to grow? What kind of soil do these herbs need? What is the best location for your herbal garden? How do you store your herbs after harvesting them? There are so many factors you might be overwhelmed at first but worry not; this chapter will be here to guide you.

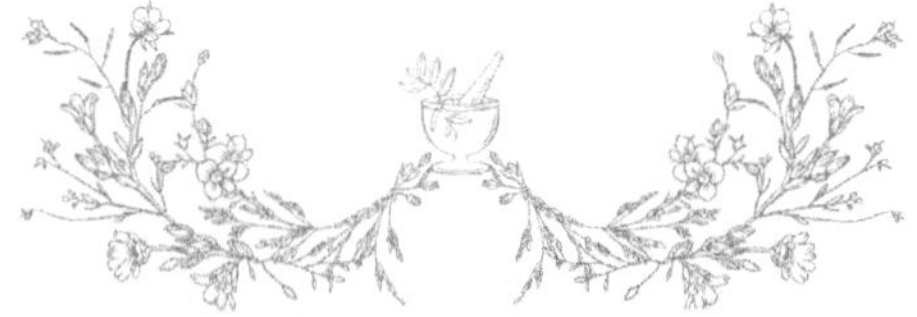

Knowing The Growing Essentials First

Planning is the first thing to be executed. However, to do this efficiently, you must equip yourself with vital knowledge about herbalism and basic herbal gardening tricks at home. You can begin by listing what herbs best suit your garden's condition. Take great care with researching the herbs you want and what fits best in your location. The previous chapter in this book can provide a great starting point.

Remember that plants grow in entirely different environments; it takes vigilance to keep them thriving. For instance, clove and ginger will grow well in tropical regions, but hemp will not thrive under those conditions.

Similarly, growth conditions, cultivation, and appropriate harvest time are critical in ensuring that your herbal garden becomes successful. Knowing the most suitable time to grow and harvest your herbs is necessary because you want your plants to stay alive so that you can maximize their health benefits.

Notice how different herbs provide herbal actions? These are possible because of the compounds that reside in specific plant parts. Failure to get your plants to grow in the best conditions severely compromises the number of active compounds that your plants develop.

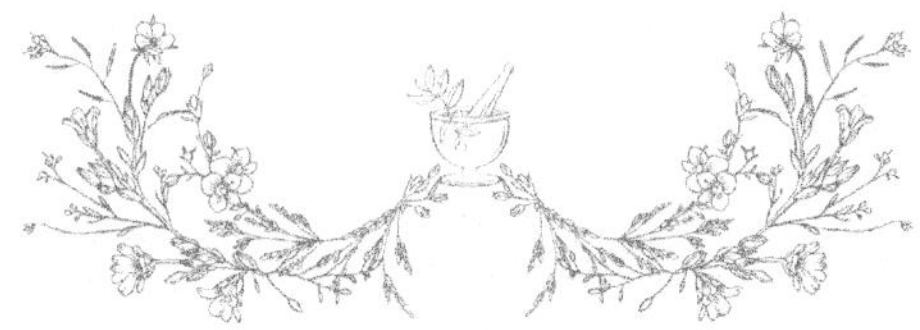

Growing Is Magical!

The steps directly involved in growing your plant are where the magic happens. However, you need to be equipped first with information about cultivation, tilling, and other factors that will impact the growth of your herbs.

Proper cultivating and tilling will give you the best results for your herbal garden. Sometimes the two words are used interchangeably, but they have some differences. Cultivation commonly refers to manipulating soil to make it appropriate for planting seedlings or other plant parts *(Carter & Mckyes, 2005)*. It can also include removing weeds, loosening the earth, or adding organic materials.

On the other hand, tilling pertains to a broader idea, including soil modification, putting the correct fertilizer, and even working on the constraint in growth due to weather and soil *(Carter & Mckyes, 2005)*. Hence, tilling is geared toward improving the soil's structure and quality to ensure the plant's growth and nourishment.

The right location will pair well with proper cultivation and tilling. Know that particular herbs prefer a certain amount of sunlight exposure, water, and soil type. Think of these elements when determining what herbs will thrive in the space that you have allocated to your garden.

Growing your herbal garden does not always need to be outdoors. Indoor gardening is an option you can try. This method allows you to set up a corner of your home for pots and containers filled with amazing herbs. Just make sure to use sterilized soil to reduce the presence of weeds and pests. The downside here is that sterilized soil does not have many of the natural nutrients you would find outside, so you may need to add fertilizer periodically.

Indoor gardening can sometimes cut off the sunlight exposure needed by some herbs. Parsley, chives, and thyme need loads of sunlight. To compensate, try setting up supplemental light using LED bulbs.

If you have the space for outdoor growing, then go for it! You can plant an in-ground garden, aerial, or container garden. Sometimes, outdoor areas like porches and decks can make up for the inadequacies of indoor gardening.

For the soil quality of outdoor growing, you will have more options and versatility. Generally, outdoor garden soil is already good enough to nourish most herbs. However, if you find your herb wilting due to the inadequacy of the soil, try making up for it by using compost.

Healthy soil has a well-balanced combination of sand, organic matter, air, water, and clay. When you ensure that your plants are nourished, watered sufficiently, and kept in areas with a decent amount of sunlight, you can grow your herbal garden in no time!

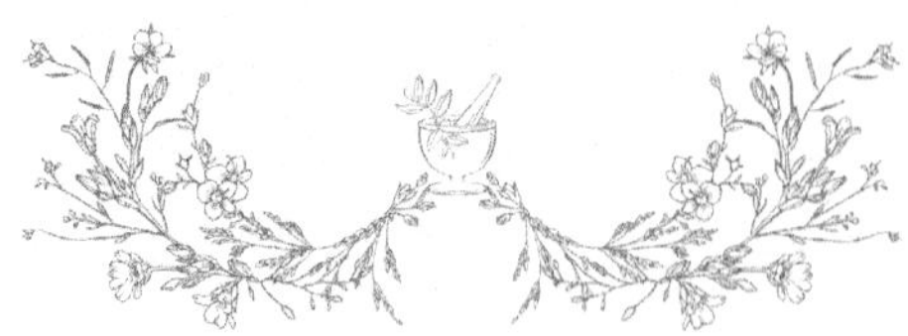

Harvesting: The Most Exciting Part

Your hard work and devoted time growing your herb will pay off after a successful harvest. As easy as it may sound, harvesting holds more thought than merely picking plant parts. Remember that proper harvesting is another vital aspect that ensures that your herbs give you optimum medicinal benefits.

Before you get to harvesting, make sure that you have your equipment on hand. Your tools do not necessarily need to be fancy, but they must be appropriate for the job. You can choose to use herb snips, hand pruners, or even your fingertips *(Jabbour, 2021).* When harvesting large amounts of woody herbs like rosemary, hand pruners are most appropriate for the job. You can use herb snips for slender herbs, or if you only need small portions of non-woody stems or leaves, your fingertips can get it done.

You can maximize the health benefits of your herbs if you plan your harvesting well. The optimal time of the year for harvesting depends on your herbs. As a general rule, harvest whenever an herb reaches its peak maturity. Typically, they mature during their flowering stage. Cutting herbs like basil and oregano before they flower is best since this is when their oils are at their highest *(Jabbour, 2021).* For seeds, harvest them after the flowers have just matured and dried. If you are only picking some herbs for additional flavor to your dishes, gathering them anytime is fine, as long as you use them immediately.

Flowers also hold herbal benefits, so it is best to harvest them during their bud stage. Unfortunately, pollinated flowers are not the most optimal since they already have depreciated qualities. Leaves are harvested best before they bud, and roots are generally harvested during autumn. Lastly, for fruits and berries, collect them as they ripen. These are only general ideas, and it all depends on the condition and climate of your garden.

The time of the day also matters. Collecting herbs in the morning after sunrise is ideal because the dew over your garden has usually evaporated during this time *(Jabbour, 2021).* Also, your herbs will have immense flavor during the early morning because the afternoon heat evaporates their flavorful oils. Only harvest the amount you need. Gathering more will only lead to excessive stress on your garden. Proper storage should be your next priority when picking herb parts for further extraction or processing.

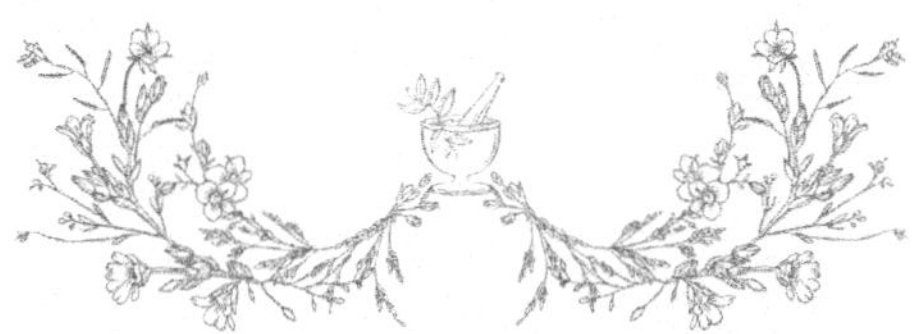

Do Not Neglect Storage

You do not want to have soggy plant parts hanging around your kitchen. Maximizing their freshness can be achieved with proper storage. Herbs usually depreciate due to excess moisture, too much sun exposure, and extra oxygen after you harvest them *(Rana, 2017).* Whether you have fresh or dried whole herbs, or leaves and powders, all herbs depreciate fast if you do not keep an eye on their shelf life.

In allocating a pantry for your herbs, ensure that it is away from excessive sunlight and moisture. Also, after thoroughly drying your herbs, leave them whole until you intend to use them. I have a wall in my pantry that I pin and hang my whole herbs on, but some herbs do not hang well. For those, you need to store them in airtight containers. Do not forget to label everything with its harvest dates.

Soft herbs like cilantro, mint and basil should have their base stems snipped and any discolored branches removed when storing your fresh herbs. You will want to place them in a jar with about an inch of water. Seal them with an airtight lid, and store them in your refrigerator. Rosemary, thyme, and other hard herbs should be wrapped in a damp loose paper towel before putting them in zip-lock bags or any airtight container. These methods help keep the plant's optimum moisture.

Appropriate storage of your herbs makes your apothecary neat and preserves the health benefits locked inside your precious herbs. After growing, harvesting, and storing your herbs, you can take your herbal journey to the next level by stocking your apothecary with homemade herbal formulas.

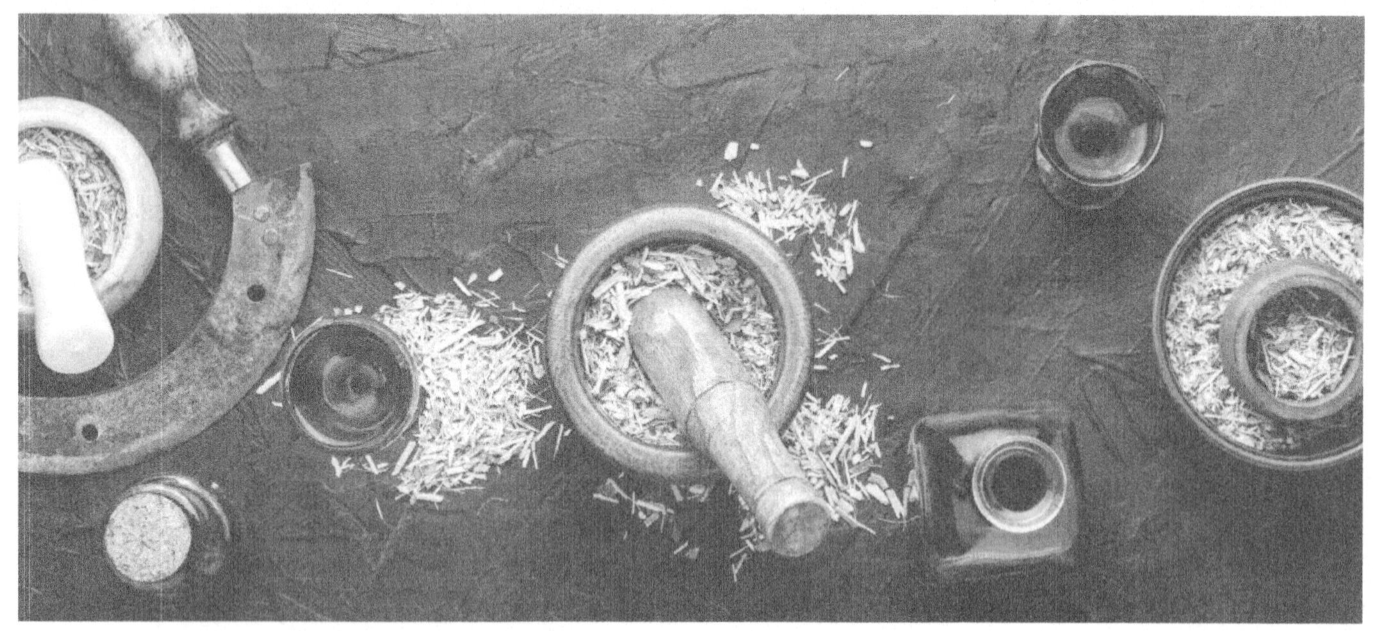

Chapter 8

Homemade Apothecary Preparation Techniques in 5 Steps or Less

After studying the previous chapters, the next step is to prepare your herbs to maximize their active compounds. In this chapter, we will look into herbal preparations you can easily do at home. As a recommendation, use stainless steel tools whenever possible. Plastic tools are not recommended, especially for formulas made with hot liquids. So, prepare your tools and herbs and follow these easy steps to create homemade remedies!

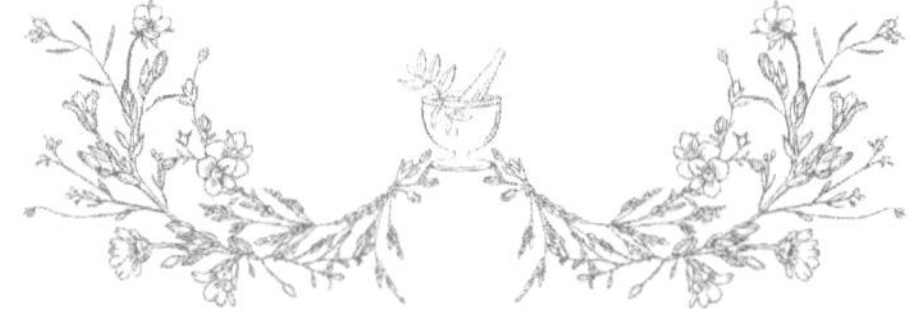

Infusions (Hot & Cold)

Brewing yourself a cup of tea is already a form of herbal preparation. Infused mixtures of flowers, stems, and leaves can be a soothing drink or can be used on external needs like compresses for bumps or scrapes. Infusions can be prepared either hot or cold, and you should keep in mind the ratio of water to the herb. This way, you get the optimal benefits in your brewed concoction. The balance can differ depending on what herbs you are using and what plant parts are being brewed. This way, you get the optimal benefits in your brewed concoction.

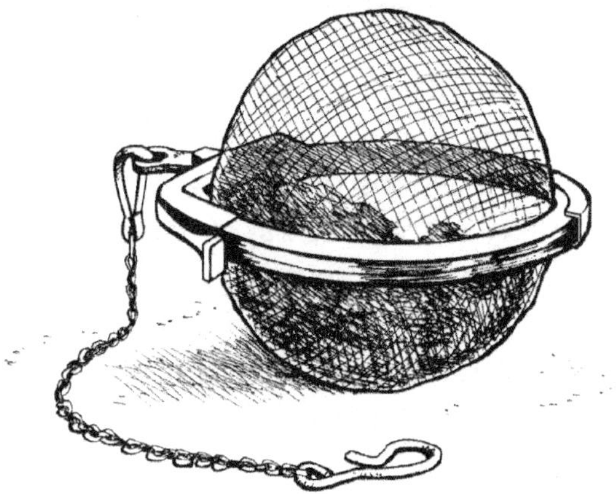

Things you will need:
1. Tea infuser or tea ball
2. Teapot or mug
3. Loose leaf or other herbs and plants of choice (or a blend)
4. Kettle (especially for hot infusion)

Preparation:

Hot Infusion
1. Place the appropriate amount of herbs in a strainer or tea infuser ball.
2. Fill your mug or container with freshly boiled water.
3. Place the strainer or tea ball in your mug or container and cover.
4. TIME YOUR TEA! Steep for around 1–10 minutes, depending on what herbs you use, then remove your tea infuser. If you desire, add a teaspoon of honey to sweeten.

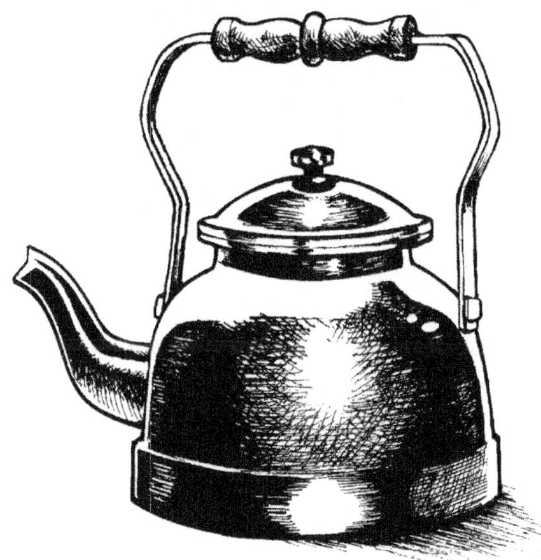

Cold Infusion

Cold infusion makes use of virtually the same steps as hot infusions. Just make sure to use water that is cold or at room temperature. Then, steep your herb for four to eight hours and strain.

If you intend to use ice when you drink this remedy, double the amount of herbs, so the flavor does not get watered down.

Pot or Kettle Infusion

1. Warm up your pot and add the desired herb.
2. Pour boiling water into the pot, put the lid on, and steep for NO MORE than 10 minutes. (Depends on the herbs used)
3. Strain into a cup. You can use a separate filter or a teapot with a built-in strainer.

Tips & Tricks

Quantity in a Cup (hot or cold): About 1 teaspoon (about 2 grams) dried herbs or about 2 teaspoons (about 4 grams) fresh herbs to 1 cup (about 8 ⅓ ounces) of water equals one dose

Quantity in a Pot: About ¼ cup (20 grams) dried herbs or about ½ cup (30 grams) fresh herbs to 2 cups (about 16 ⅔ ounces) of water

Dosage: Drink about 2 cups (500 milliliters) three to four times a day

Storage: Store in a covered container in the refrigerator or cool place for no longer than 24 hours.

Decoctions

Decoctions and infusions are both herbal formulas that use water as their extracting solvent. Essentially, decoctions are made by simmering tough herb parts like roots, dried berries, seeds, or barks. This preparation produces a more concentrated tea with a more robust flavor *(Kendle, 2018).* You have the option to take decoctions hot or cold.

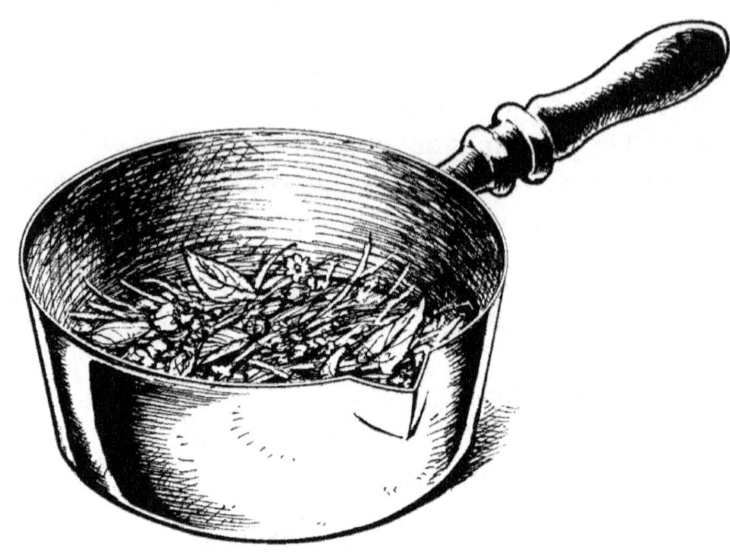

Things you will need:

1. Your herbs or plants of choice (or a blend)
2. Small saucepan and a stove
3. Jar or container

Preparation:

1. Place your desired amount of herbs and about a quart of water in a small saucepan. Bring it to a simmer for 20–45 minutes. The liquid will reduce about a third as you simmer your decoction.
2. After your decoction is simmered, strain it into a separate jar or container. Drink a cup now, and

store the remaining decoction in a cool place.

Tips & Tricks

Quantity: About ¼ cup (20 grams) of dried herbs or ¾ cup (40 grams) of fresh herbs to 3 cups (750 milliliters) of cold water. It will reduce to about 2 cups (500 milliliters) after simmering, equaling 3–4 doses.

Dosage: Take 2 cups (500 milliliters) three to four times daily

Storage: Store in a covered container in the refrigerator or cool place for no longer than 48 hours.

Tinctures

Tinctures typically use alcohol as the solvent to release the beneficial compounds in plants. Generally, tinctures are potent, fast-acting, and have a long shelf life. The ratio of herb to solvent classifies them, and your finished product should be at least 20% alcohol (40 proof) to ensure it is shelf-stable. Recommendations are to use 80–90 proof vodka for most plant parts. Gums and resins will need a higher concentration, usually 190 proof. To ensure suitable alcohol concentrations, research the herbs and plant parts you use.

⚠ **Cautions:** Do not use rubbing alcohol, industrial alcohols, or methyl alcohol. Do not use alcohol when pregnant or experiencing gastric inflammation; use apple cider vinegar or glycerol for nonalcoholic tinctures.

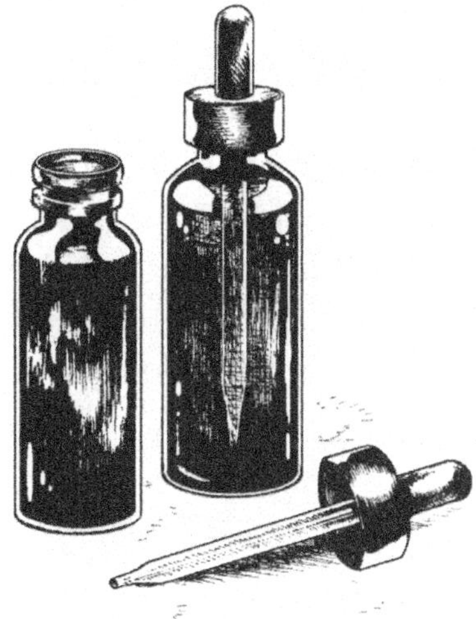

Things you will need:

1. Your herbs or plants of choice (or a blend) CHOPPED
2. Vodka (vinegar or glycerol)
3. Large pot or wine press (if you use a wine press, you will need a small pitcher to catch the liquid)
3. Large glass jar with a lid
4. Parchment paper
5. Cheesecloth or wire strainer
6. Funnel
7. Dark glass bottles with corks or screw-on caps

Preparation:

1. Place your herbs in a large dry glass jar and pour alcohol over them. Make sure to submerge your herbs into at least two inches (about five centimeters) of liquid. Alcohol may affect the rubber seal

of your container, so place parchment paper between your jar and its lid.

2. Seal and label your jar. Shake your tincture well for a couple of minutes before storing it in a cool dark place for 10–14 days. Every day or two, take it out and shake it up nicely for a minute or two.

3. When it is time to strain, place cheesecloth or strainer over the top of a large pot or wine press. If you use a wine press, push down to squeeze your tincture into a small pitcher. If you use a large pot, pour your mixture over the cheesecloth, bring the sides together, then twist and squeeze the herbs until all the liquid is removed. Alternatively, you can use a fine-mesh strainer over a large bowl and a smaller bowl to press the mixture.

4. Take your prepared tincture and pour it into clean dark glass bottles using a funnel. Close the bottles with corks or screw-on caps. Label with "date prepared" and herbs used. Store in a cool dark place.

Tips & Tricks

Quantity: Generally, use 1-part fresh herbs to 2-parts liquid (1:2 ratio), or for dried herbs, use a 1:5 ratio. Chop your herbs into small pieces and add them to the alcohol. Using vodka (35–40% alcohol) is ideal, but rum can be used as an alternative to mask the taste of unpleasant or bitter herbs.

Dosage: Dilute one teaspoon (five milliliters) of tincture in about 1.5 tablespoons (25 milliliters) of water or juice and take two to three times daily.

Storage: Ideally, stored in clean, dark-colored glass bottles. Store somewhere cool, dark, and dry for around two years.

Infused Oils

Infused oils are herbal preparations produced using carrier oils applied to dried or chopped fresh plant parts. Two variations – hot or cold oils – are solutions with many therapeutic effects. You can use these for bug bites, minor burns or cuts, and skin care oil for dry lips. They can also be added to ointments and creams to use for massages. Infused oils are not the same as essential oils. Essential oils contain active ingredients naturally found in plants, but you can add them to infused oils to increase the remedy's potency.

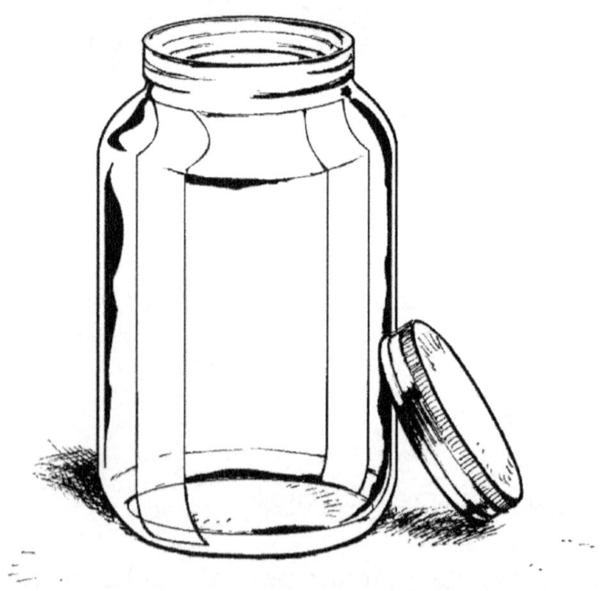

Things you will need:
1. Your herbs or plants of choice (or a blend), dried or coarsely chopped
2. Oil (sunflower oil, avocado oil, or olive oil works best)
3. Glass bowl (heat resistant) that fits nicely over a saucepan
4. Saucepan (medium)
5. Jar or wine press
6. Muslin bag (cheesecloth or nylon mesh will do as well)
7. Funnel
8. Dark glass bottle with a cork or screw-on top

Preparation:

Hot Infused Oils

1. Using your glass bowl, mix your chopped herbs and oil. Fill a saucepan about halfway with water and bring to a boil. Set the chopped herbs and oil bowl on top and reduce the heat to low. Cover and simmer for two to three hours. You can also use a double boiler in place of the heat resistance bowl and saucepan.
2. Remove your mixture from the heat and let it cool. After cooling, proceed to strain the mixture in a wine press. If you do not have a wine press, use a muslin bag over a jar or bowl to strain, then squeeze out the oils.
3. Pour your infused oil into a dark glass bottle and seal with a cork or screw-on top. Label with "date prepared" and herbs used. Store in a cool dark place.

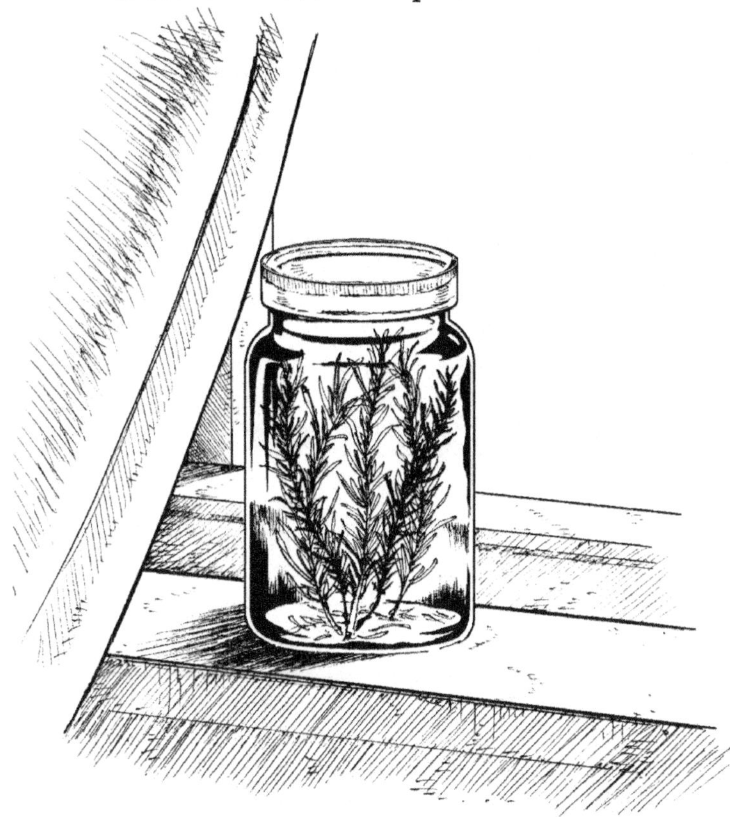

Cold Infused Oils

1. Pour your oil over your chopped herbs in a clear glass jar. Submerge your herbs in oil entirely and shake well. Place your preparation on a sunny windowsill for two to six weeks.
2. Insert your mixture through a muslin bag over a large mouth jar or pitcher. Make sure the bag hangs with space to allow the oil to drip filter into the bottom of the container. Continue straining

by squeezing the remaining oils from the herbs in the bag.

3. Pour your infused oil into a dark glass bottle and seal with a cork or screw-on top. Label with "date prepared" and herbs used. Store in a cool dark place.

Tips & Tricks

Quantity: About 2 ¼ cups (250 grams) of dried herbs or 9 ¼ cups (500 grams) of fresh herbs to about three cups (750 milliliters) of choice oil (high-quality avocado, sunflower, or olive oil).

Dosage: Unless otherwise prescribed by a doctor, you can use and consume as much as you want!

Storage: Store in a clean, airtight, dark glass container for upwards of a year. If you want the best results, use your preparation within six months.

Essential Oils

Essential oils are sometimes confused with the previously explored infused oils. These two have very different methods of preparation. All essential oils are made with steam distillation, but these high-quality and commercially-made products can get quite expensive.

I was apprehensive about making essential oils at home for a long time. Once I finally tried it myself, I found it was not as complicated as I thought! If you want to try making your essential oils, here are some simple steps to follow.

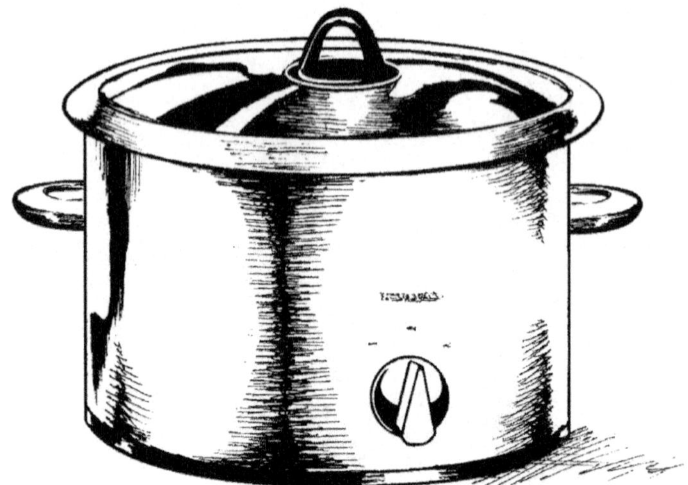

Things you will need:

1. CHOPPED FRESH plant part of choice (make sure it can fill more than half of your crockpot)
2. Distilled water
3. Crockpot
4. Turkey Baster
5. Small dark glass bottles with screw-on caps

Preparation:

1. Put about 3–4 cups (165–215 grams) of CHOPPED FRESH plant parts in the crockpot and cover it with water. Water must be no more than ¾ of your crockpot's volume. Place your lid UPSIDE DOWN so that steam condensation will drop back into your pot. You can also use a plate if it fits your crockpot size.
2. Turn your crockpot on high. After the water reaches a hot temperature (not boiling), switch it to low and simmer for 3–4 hours.

3. After, turn off the heat and set aside to COOL COMPLETELY before placing it in a refrigerator overnight.
4. The next day, you will notice a thin film over the top. This film is your essential oil. It will be somewhat hardened, and you must gather the substance quickly before it falls away as the crockpot warms up to room temperature. Lift the oils out of the water using a turkey baster, doing your best not to gather water in the process. You can always reheat the essential oil after the first gathering if you accidentally collect some water. BE CAREFUL and do not overdo it if you choose to reheat because essential oils lose their potency when heated.
5. Pour into a dark bottle, and seal with an airtight screw-on top. Label with "date prepared" and herbs used. Store in a cool dark place.

Tips & Tricks

Dosage for massage: Always use carrier oil with your essential oil, whether you make your own or buy them commercially. You can use one essential oil or choose two or three to create a blend. Mix 5–10 drops to one tablespoon of carrier oil, such as grape seed oil, and gently massage the skin.

Dosage in an oil diffuser: A great way to relax and enjoy your essential oils is to burn them in a diffuser. You can make a blend of more than one, but it is not recommended to use more than three. Put 5–10 drops in and let it burn for 30 minutes at a time. Leaving a diffuser on longer is not recommended.

Storage: Store in dark glass containers in a cool dark place for upwards of a year. They start to lose potency at about six months, so utilize them accordingly.

Tonic Wines

Tonic wines give us herbal preparations that are very close to herbal teas. These are both easily consumed concoctions that help us utilize the benefits of herbs to improve our health. Making tonic wines involves carefully selecting different plant parts. Some common herbs and plant parts are angelica root, fennel seed, cassia bark, mugwort, cardamom seeds, coriander seed, and peppermint leaves.

Oxygen is detrimental to a potent, safe tonic wine. When the air gets to the herbs, it can mold them and make the tonic wine ineffective and unsafe. Therefore, I do not recommend using jars. Instead, a dark glass jug with a tap at the bottom is the best solution for limiting exposure to air.

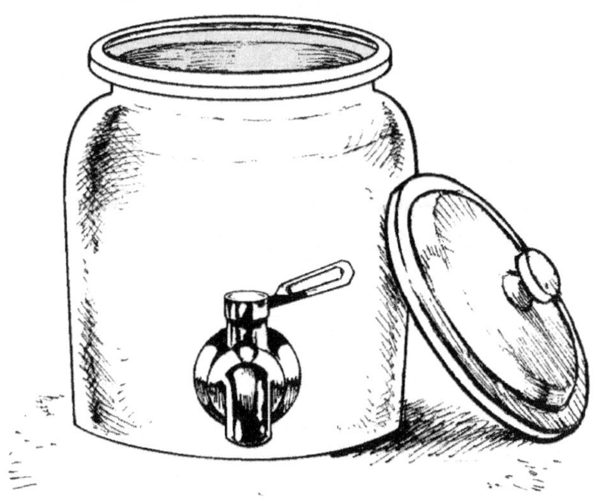

Things you will need:

1. Your choice of tonic or bitter plant parts (or a blend)
2. Red or white wine
3. Dark glass or ceramic jug with a tap at the bottom

Preparation:

1. Place herbs in the bottom of a dry, clean jug.
2. Cover herbs completely with choice wine and seal the jug with an airtight lid.
3. Label with "date prepared" and herbs used. Store in a cool dark place.
4. Infuse the solution for a minimum of two weeks or a maximum of six weeks. Cheers!

Tips & Tricks

Quantity: About 1 ⅛ cup (100 grams) dried tonic herbs, or about 3 ⅔ cups (200 grams) fresh tonic herbs, or about ¼ cup (25 grams) dried bitter herbs to about 1 liter (1 quart) of choice wine.

Dosage: Take about ½ cup (70 milliliters) every day before a meal

Storage: Store in a dark glass jug for 3–4 months. Add wine as needed to keep the herbs covered completely, but do your best to limit the exposure to air. If the plant matter starts to mold, discard the tonic immediately as it becomes unsafe for drinking.

Syrups

If you want to explore herbal preparations on the sweeter side, herbal syrups are an excellent choice. Syrups are made by mixing a sweetener, usually honey or unrefined sugar, into decoctions or infusions. Sweeteners can extend the shelf life of these herbal preparations.

This preparation is incredible for relieving sore throats and makes an excellent vehicle for cough mixtures. Since it is sweet, it can mask the taste of unpleasant herbs, making it perfect for children! You can also mix herbal syrups into your favorite cocktails to add an exciting layer of flavor.

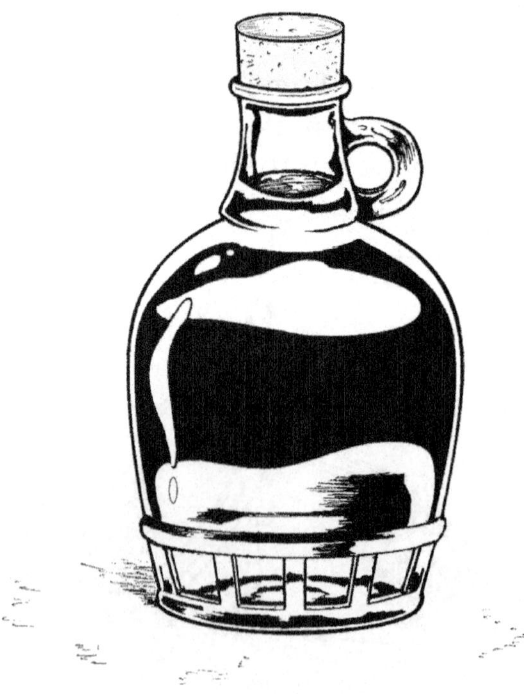

Things you will need:
1. Saucepan and stove
2. Decoction or infusion (previously prepared with choice herbs and plants)
3. Sugar or sweetener of choice (honey, maple syrup, glycerin, etc.)
4. Funnel
5. Dark glass bottle with a cork stopper

Preparation:
1. Pour your decoction or infusion into a saucepan and add the desired sweetener. For infusions, you will want to simmer at low heat for a maximum of 15 minutes. If you choose to use a decoction, you need to simmer it for no more than 30 minutes. Heat gently and continuously stir until the sugar or honey dissolves. It should have a syrup-like consistency when done.
2. Remove your saucepan from the heat and let your herbal syrup stand for around 30 minutes.
3. Transfer your syrup to a clean dark glass bottle using a funnel. Syrups tend to ferment over time and may explode if you use a screw-on cap. Instead, use a cork stopper to avoid any dangerous and sticky mishaps.
4. Label with "date prepared" and herbs used. Store in a cool dark place.

Tips & Tricks

Quantity: About 2 cups (500 milliliters) infusion or decoction, infused or heated for the maximum time depending on which you choose; about 1 ½ cups (500 grams) of choice sweetener. My personal favorite is local raw honey! If you use dry sweeteners, like unrefined sugar, use about 2 ½ cups because they are lighter in weight.

Dosage: Take about 1–2 teaspoons (5–10 milliliters) no more than three times a day

Storage: Stored best in sterile dark glass bottles with a cork stopper. Keep your syrups in a cool and dark place for no longer than six months.

Ointments & Salves

Ointments are herbal preparations made with oils or fats but have no water component. They can be made with many different bases, such as beeswax, olive oil, coconut oil, petroleum jelly, or a combination of oils. Note that using different types of bases will yield different consistencies. Using beeswax will give your ointment a relatively solid texture, while using petroleum jelly will be less firm.

The great thing about ointments is they provide a protective layer between the skin and the outside environment. They are gentle on the skin but very effective. They can nourish your skin and boost its ability to absorb nutrients. Ointments are applied topically on scrapes, itchy or dry skin, hemorrhoids, and rashes, including diaper rash. Here is an easy beeswax salve recipe I use to replace all of my store-bought ointments.

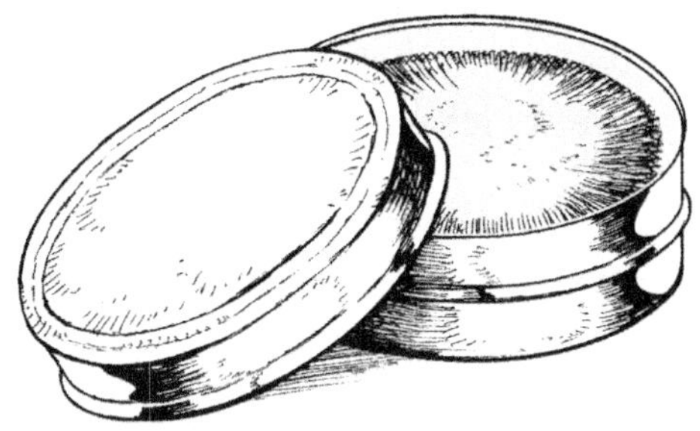

Things you will need:
1. FINELY CHOPPED choice herbs and plants (or a blend)
2. Choice of edible oil (sweet almond or grape seed)
3. Shea butter or Cocoa butter
4. Beeswax
5. Choice of essential oil (optional)
6. Jelly bag and string
7. Wide mouth jug or pitcher
8. Rubber kitchen gloves
9. Containers with lids (wide-mouth jars or tins work great!)
10. Double boiler (or heat-resistant bowl and saucepan)

Preparation:
1. Combine choice oil, shea or cocoa butter, and beeswax in a double boiler. To improvise, a heat-resistant bowl placed over a saucepan will also work.
2. Add your chopped herbs to the melted oil and simmer as you continuously stir for 15 minutes.
3. Secure a jelly bag (cheesecloth, muslin bag, or even old tights will work) to a wide-mouth jug or pitcher with a string.
4. Pour oil through the jelly bag and allow it to filter through. You can extract more oils by squeezing the bag. It can be hot, so make sure to use protective rubber gloves.
5. It is optional to add a few drops of choice essential oil at this point. Stir to combine the melted components and immediately pour them into your container. Be quick before the ointment starts to solidify! Once it has cooled completely, tighten the lid and label it for later use.

Tips & Tricks

Quantity: About ½ cup (45 grams) dried or about 2 ¼ cups (286 grams) fresh herbs or plant parts (or a blend) to 1/2 cup (60 grams) beeswax; 1/2 cup (60 grams) cocoa butter or shea butter; 1 cup EDIBLE oil of choice. You can choose to use about ¼ cup (22.5 grams) of dried powdered herbs to avoid having to strain. (Add more beeswax if your ointment is too thin, or add more oil if your ointment is too thick.)

Dosage: Apply topically to the affected area three times a day. For diaper rashes, apply ointment after every diaper change.

Storage: Stores nicely in a clean wide-mouth jar or tin with a tight lid for about three months.

Creams

Herbal creams nourish and can soothe dry, damaged, or dull skin. The effects of creams are due to a combination of the active compounds of the herbs added and the moisturizing capability of shea butter and oils. Creating creams using your homegrown herbs is an enjoyable process!

Like ointments, creams are prepared with oil or fat but emulsified in water. The process is similar to ointments, although the water can separate if you rush. Here is an all-time favorite recipe I use for a massage cream. My clients love how it makes their skin feel and does not leave an oily residue like some ointments.

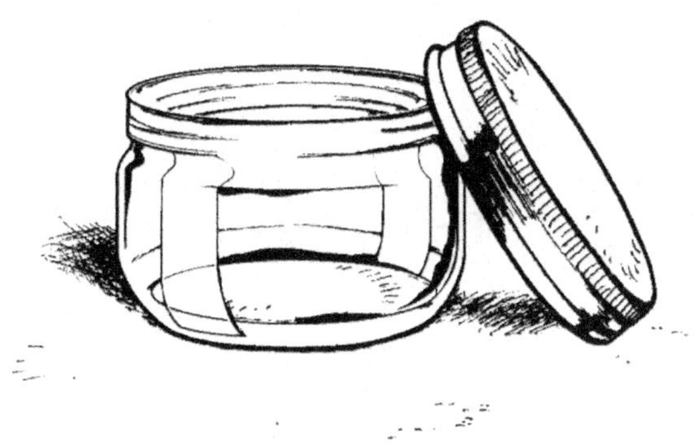

Things you will need:
1. Your herb or plant parts of choice (or a blend)
2. Distilled water
3. Shea butter (you can also use emulsifying wax)
4. Glycerine
5. Double boiler or a heat-resistant bowl over a saucepan
6. Wide mouth jug or pitcher
7. Jelly bag (cheesecloth or muslin bag will work)
8. Small knife or cake spatula
9. Dark-colored jars; wide-mouthed jars with screw-on lids

Preparation:
1. Melt your shea butter in a heat-resistant bowl over a saucepan of boiling water, or use a double boiler. After it melts, add glycerine, distilled water, and your herbs or plant parts.
2. Bring it to a gentle simmer for 3 hours.
3. After 3 hours, secure a jelly bag over a clean jug or pitcher to strain out the plant parts. SLOWLY and continuously stir your preparation until it sets.
4. Once your cream is set, you can use a small knife or cake spatula to pack it in dark glass jars with screw-on lids. Label with the herb used and "date prepared" and store for later use.

Tips & Tricks

Quantity: About ⅓ cup (30 grams) dried or about 1 ⅓ cups (75 grams) fresh herbs; about ⅔ cup (150 grams) shea butter (or emulsifying wax); about ¼ cup (70 grams) glycerine; about ½ cup (80 milliliters) distilled water

Dosage: Apply immediately to dry skin after you shower to lock in moisture while your pores are open. Reapply up to three times a day.

Storage: Stores nicely in a clean, airtight dark glass jar in the refrigerator for around three months.

Poultices

Poultices have been used for centuries for their exceptional healing properties. They can help with inflammation caused by nerves, broken bones, sprains, strains, and muscle pain. A poultice can draw out the infection if you have a pus-infected wound, like an ulcer or boil.

Poultices are a paste-like preparation usually applied directly to the skin and held with a moist warm cloth. I used a poultice after long hikes, especially the first one of the spring. I do not do much hiking during the winter months, and my calves tend to tighten and spasm after my first hike of the spring season.

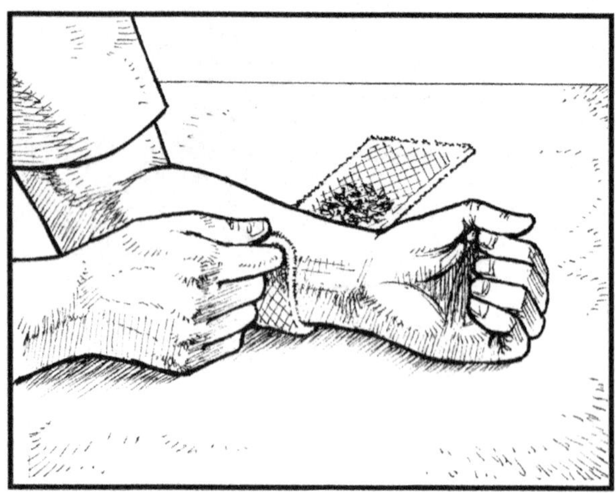

Things you will need:
1. Your herb of choice, finely chopped or crushed into powder
2. Coconut oil
3. Distilled water
4. Saucepan
5. Bandage or clean cheesecloth

Preparation:
1. In a saucepan, simmer your herbs in distilled water for around two minutes.
2. Pour herbs over cheesecloth and squeeze out any excess liquid.
3. Using a bandage or a clean cheesecloth, secure the processed herb over your desired area. You can apply oil over your skin first to prevent the plant parts from sticking. I like to make a pouch with cheesecloth and wrap the affected area with an ace bandage to secure it because you need to leave a poultice in place for up to 3 hours. Do not wrap it too tight because you still want blood flow to get to the area.

Tips & Tricks

Quantity: Use as many herbs as you need to cover the affected area. The larger the area, the more herbs you will need.

Dosage: Apply a poultice as needed for at least three hours. You can repeat this process as many times as you need to.

Storage: Poultices should always be made fresh for every application.

Compresses

Compresses are a simple topical herbal application to manage muscle soreness or inflammation due to skin bumps or bruises. Essentially, compresses use a clean cloth soaked in herbal infusions, decoctions, or tinctures and then placed on the area of concern.

I like to use compresses when I do not feel like spending time on a poultice. I usually have a tincture for inflammation and can quickly apply a compress to relieve inflammatory pain. Cold compresses are beneficial for headaches and cooling fevers. I also find hot and cold compresses pleasant to use for massage clients, as they are quick and easy.

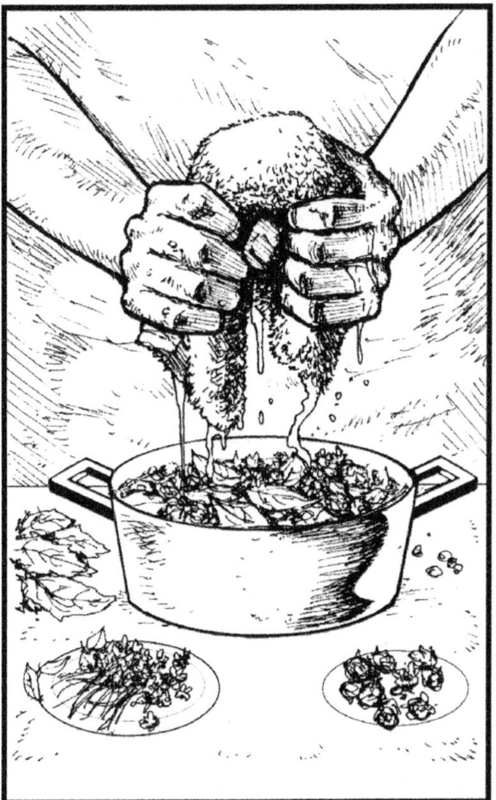

Things you will need:
1. Strong herbal tea of choice (infusion, decoction, or DILUTED tincture)
2. Clean cloth (at least two)
3. Glass bowl
4. Safety pins

Preparation:
1. Make sure you have clean hands before utilizing compresses. You can opt to apply some oil on the area of concern to prevent the compress from sticking and for a less messy experience. Soak a clean piece of soft cloth in a bath of strong herbal tea. Wring out the excess liquid.
2. Place your soaked cloth on your affected area. Cover it with a dry cloth or plastic wrap to hold it in place, and secure it with a safety pin.
3. Leave it on for one to two hours.

Tips & Tricks

Infusion or Decoction Quantity: About 2 cups (500 milliliters)

Tincture Quantity: About 5 teaspoons (25 milliliters) to 2 cups (500 milliliters) of distilled water

Dosage: Apply lotion compress as needed. Always make a new hot preparation after it cools. If you have a cold compress, create a new one once the cloth is dry.

Storage: Prepared lotions are stored nicely in a clean bottle with a lid inside the refrigerator for up to two days.

Pills, Powders, & Capsules

One of the most common forms of herbal products that you might see is pills or capsules. You can easily make these at home using your herbal apothecary. This process will save you loads of money and ensure you consume only the freshest organic ingredients. Just be very careful about the kind of herb and dosage you put in them. Do your research!

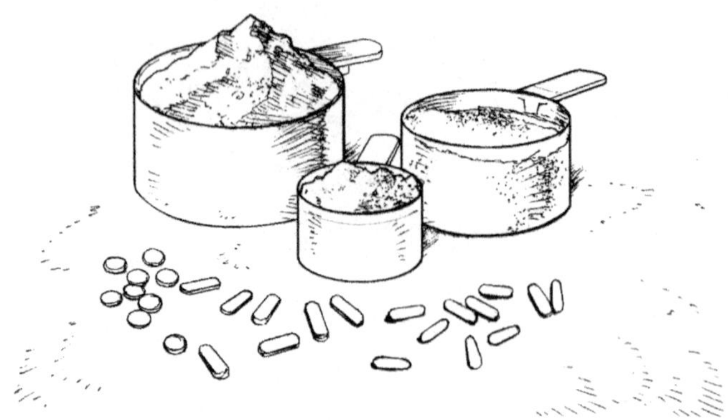

Things you will need:

1. Powdered organic herb
2. Empty capsules (gelatin, HPMC, or Pullulan capsules work well)
3. Capsule machine, a.k.a capsule tray (optional)
4. A small dish
5. Dark glass jar with a screw-on top

Manual Capsule Preparation:

1. Pour herb or plant powder into a small dish and position the empty sides of the capsule halves toward each other, open side inward. Scoop up the powder into each half.
2. When full of power, gently slide the two halves together and do your best not to spill the powder. This process can be tricky the first time, but with practice, it becomes easier. You can also use a capsule machine to produce a lot in a small amount of time.

Preparation With a Capsule Machine:

1. Position your empty capsules in the capsule machine. Carefully measure your powdered herb and use it to fill your capsules. You can use your capsule machine's spreader to help distribute your powdered herbs evenly into the capsules.
2. Press down on the machine to pack the herb powder into your capsules. Make sure to alternate between the tamping device and the spreader to complete the encapsulation process.

Pill Preparation:

Another noteworthy option is the use of herbal pills. These are similar to capsules; however, these pills do not have an external coating. You may see pills or tablets in different shapes, but these are designed to contain a specific amount of powder.

The trick with pills is using another ingredient to hold the powdered herbs together. You can make your pills by combining honey with powdered herbs to achieve a dough-like consistency. Then, roll it into a small snake-like roll and cut according to the desired dose. It is optional to roll your small herbal pills in cinnamon or cocoa powder before storing them in a cool, dark, and dry place.

Tips & Tricks

Quantity: Fill your capsules (size 00) with about 250 milligrams of powdered herbs or plant parts

Dosage: Take two or three capsules twice a day. Sometimes best taken with food depending on the plant you use.

Storage: Stores nicely in an airtight dark glass jar kept in a cool, dry, and dark place for up to three or four months.

Bath & Skin Washes

Bathing your skin in soothing herbal solutions can help rejuvenate your skin and relax tense muscles. They are also great for clearing out stuffy noses. Baths and skin washes are enjoyable to experiment with, so have fun with them! Let's explore two options.

Things you will need:

1. Your herb of choice (either fresh or dried)
2. Distilled water
3. Soap of choice
4. Essential oil or infused oils are optional
5. Mortar and pestle
6. Grater
7. Saucepan
8. Bathtub (if you are soaking)

Soap Skin Wash Preparation:

1. Grind your herbs in a mortar and pestle to achieve a paste-like or powdery consistency. You may drop a bit of distilled water to help you achieve the desired consistency.
2. Grate your chosen soap. Combine the prepared herb paste and soap in a small pan and simmer it for at least one minute to infuse the herbs. Remove your preparation from the heat and strain the herbs.
3. Let cool and apply to the affected area or the whole body in the shower and wash away thoroughly.

Bath Preparation:

1. Draw yourself a hot bath.
2. Add 2 cups (500 milliliters) of strained infusion or 5–10 drops of your favorite essential oil. You can also throw a couple of tea balls in as a substitute.
3. Soak for 15–30 minutes and repeat daily. Make sure that the water temperature is comfortable first before getting in!

Steam Inhalations

Aside from having herbal preparations made to be consumed or applied topically, you also have the option of steam inhalation. The active components of herbs are utilized by inhaling infused steam. This method may help relieve sinusitis, bronchial asthma, hay fever, or manage congested noses.

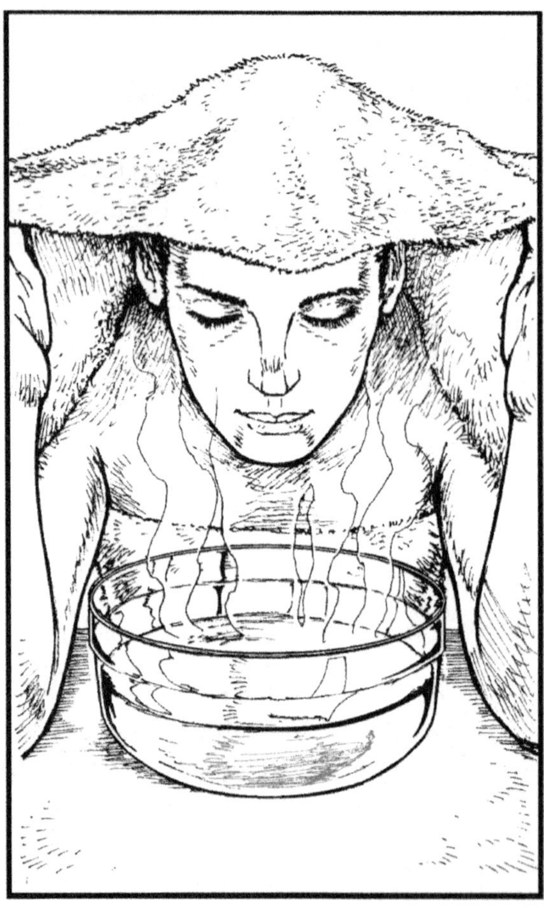

Things you will need:

1. Essential oils
2. Freshly boiled water
3. Large clean bowl
4. Large clean towel

Preparation:

1. Pour around 1 liter (1 quart) of boiled water into a large bowl.
2. Add 5–10 drops of your essential oil of choice. Eucalyptus is excellent for opening up airways. Stir it well. Cover your head and bowl with a clean towel to direct the steam upward toward your face to maximize the vapor produced.
3. You can utilize this setup for around 10 minutes. Usually, after this time, no more steam is produced. Stay in a warm room after steam inhalation to help your airways gradually adapt to a cooler temperature and help decongest the sinuses.

Tips & Tricks

Quantity: Use 1 liter (1 quart) of boiled water for every 5–10 drops of chosen essential oil or blend.
Dosage: 10–15 minute inhalation as needed for whatever sinus symptoms you may be experiencing.
Storage: Steam inhalation is always immediately used after it is prepared.

Gargles & Mouthwash

Natural mouthwash and gargles are free from other artificial ingredients like alcohol or added sweeteners. Herbal mouthwashes can also reduce harmful bacteria in the mouth that causes gum inflammation. Here is a simple recipe for your next all-natural gargle. You can use infusions, tinctures, or decoctions.

Things you will need:

1. Infusions or decoctions made from herbs with antiseptic properties

Preparation:

1. You can follow the previously mentioned steps for making an infusion or decoction.
2. Before utilizing it as mouthwash or gargle, let it rest for 15–20 minutes.
3. Proceed to swish it in the mouth, gargle, and spit completely. You may swallow this preparation if you are NOT PREGNANT.

Tips & Tricks

Quantity: ¼ cup (about 60 milliliters) of antiseptic infusion or decoction

Dosage: Swish, gargle, and spit entirely twice a day or as needed

Storage: See infusion and decoction for storage tips.

Utilizing your knowledge in herbalism and incorporating it into different preparations provides a holistic experience in your journey toward optimal vitality. The journey into herbalism allows you to control your lifestyle and reduce artificial chemicals from causing you harm. Aside from this, experimenting with your recipes and procedures is very enjoyable.

However, quality control is essential to ensure that you can truly maximize the benefits of active compounds in your herbs. Keep track of your recipes and dosages of each herb in an herbal remedies journal. Noting your preparations will help you attain a consistent result if you want to make your remedy again. Similarly, it can help you have a baseline on possible tweaks in your future recipes.

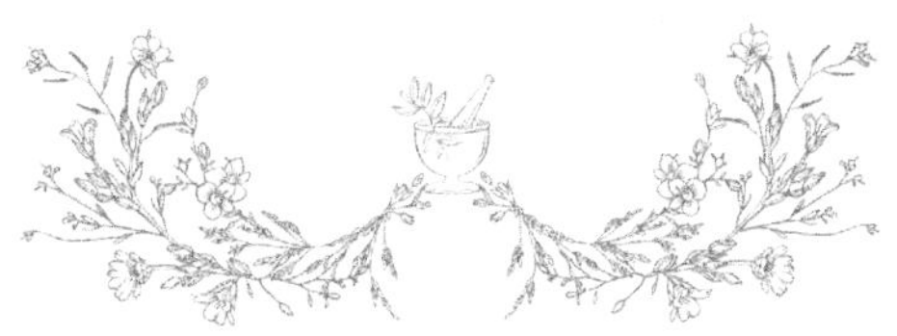

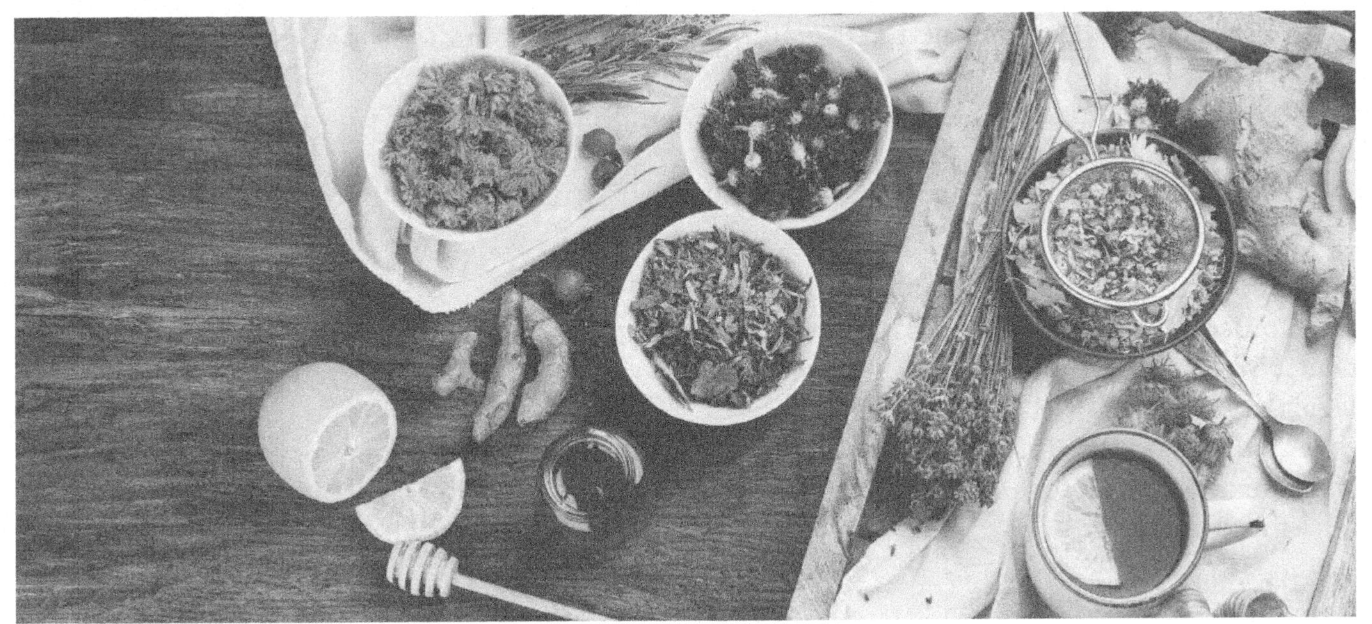

Chapter 9

Herbal Remedies for 77 Common Ailments

Having an apothecary of herbal remedies ready in the comfort of your home is crucial in maintaining a holistic lifestyle. As we have ventured along, discovering information on active components of herbs, understanding the herbs themselves, and knowing how to prepare them, you can now incorporate everything you learned to help your body recover from different common ailments.

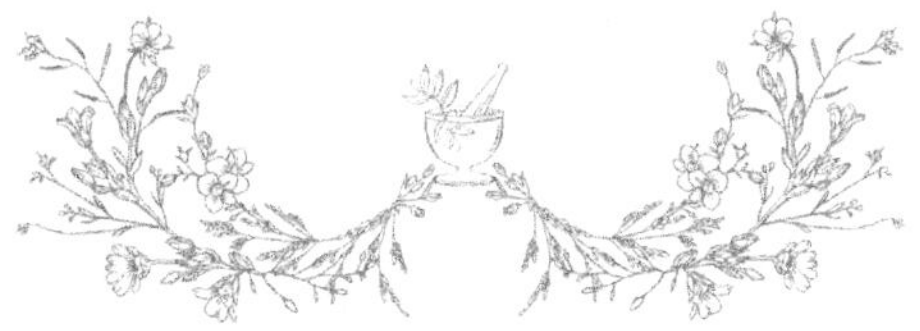

#1. Anemia
Herb: Nettle
How To Use: Infuse 25 grams of nettle into 750 milliliters of water daily
Herb: Chickweed
How to Use: Add chopped raw leaves to your dishes or blend them into sauces or dips

#2. Anxiety
Herb: Valerian

How To Use: Mix 10 drops of tincture in water; consume every hour for a maximum of two weeks
Herb: Hops
How To Use: Supplements: Take a maximum of 200 milligrams per day
Herbs: Lemon balm, Skullcap, or St. John's wort
How To Use: Prepare an infusion using any of these herbs; drink 600 milliliters daily

#3. Acne
Herb: Cinnamon
How To Use: Mix two tablespoons of honey with one teaspoon of cinnamon; apply to the face and leave it on for 10–15 minutes; rinse with water
Herb: Green Tea
How To Use: Steep the infusion for 3–4 minutes and let it cool. With a cotton pad, apply the tea to your skin and allow it to dry; rinse off excess and PAT skin dry; DO NOT rub the skin dry! (This may cause more irritation.)

#4. Allergies
Herb: Nettle or Elder
How To Use: Make an infusion or decoction with either herb and take 450–600 milliliters daily for up to three months.

#5. Arthritis (not Rheumatoid)
Herb: Aloe vera
How To Use: Take some aloe vera gel or extract fresh aloe gel from its leaves. Apply it directly to the skin around the concerned area.
Herb: Ginger and/or Turmeric
How To Use: Make an infusion and drink four cups daily until symptoms subside. Prepare a cream or ointment and apply it to the affected area three times a day for twelve weeks.

#6. Asthma
Herb: Thyme
How to Use: Infuse 15 grams in three cups of water and drink throughout the day.
Herb: Turmeric
How to Use: Make or purchase turmeric pills, powder, and capsules; take 500–2,000 milligrams daily.
Herb: Echinacea
How to Use: Use ½ teaspoon of echinacea tincture mixed with water twice daily.

#7. Athlete's foot
Herb: Turmeric and Calendula
How To Use: A mixture of ½ teaspoon turmeric powder and 15 milligrams of calendula ointment can be topically applied to feet daily.
Herb: Garlic
How To Use: Crush three to five cloves of garlic and rub over the affected part of the foot. Then let it sit for 20 minutes, wash thoroughly to remove odor, and apply up to twice daily.

#8. Backache
Herb: Thyme and/or Bay leaf
How To Use: Infuse 25 grams of leaves into three cups of water; strain infusion into hot bath; soak body for up to 20 minutes as needed.

#9. Bee sting
Herb: Aloe vera
How to Use: Apply gel or ointment topically on the affected area. (Extract the gel from fresh leaves.)
Herb: Calendula
How to Use: Make ointment, cream, OR infused oil and apply them topically as needed.
Herb: Nettle
How to Use: Mix one teaspoon tincture with water and drink three times daily for three days. (May also try infusion or decoction)

#10. Bloating
Herb: Fennel and/or Peppermint
How To Use: Infuse ¼ to ½ teaspoon of fennel seeds or peppermint in 150 milliliters of water; drink up to three cups daily.

#11. Bronchitis
Herb: Echinacea or Garlic
How To Use: Echinacea tincture — ½ teaspoon in water taken two to three times per day; OR eat two garlic cloves daily.

#12. Bruises
Herb: Arnica
How To Use: Ointment or cream applied two to three times daily (Avoid open wounds)

#13. Burns
Herb: Aloe vera gel
How To Use: Clean the burn first; apply liberally to the affected area; cover with a bandage and leave on overnight; repeat for two to three nights. ***(Immediately stop if the pain intensifies; seek professional attention for third or fourth-degree burns.)***

#14. Chapped lips
Herb: Aloe vera gel, Chamomile, Calendula, and/or Lemon Balm
How To Use: Gel, ointment, or cream applied to the lips multiple times a day; mix and match herbs or use just one (you can also make lip balm by adding more beeswax to an ointment).
Herb: Green tea
How To Use: Steep green tea bags in hot water for three to five minutes; remove bags and let cool; place over lips and leave there for a few minutes; do this once daily.

#15. Canker sores
Herb: Chamomile
How To Use: Steep a tea bag in hot water for a few minutes; remove bags and let cool; apply to the affected area and leave it on for around five minutes. After, with the brewed chamomile tea, rinse your mouth; repeat three to four times daily.
Herb: Echinacea
How To Use: Make mouthwash with one teaspoon of echinacea tincture to equal parts warm water; swish for two minutes, and SPIT OUT!

#16. Chickenpox
Herb: Echinacea and/or St. John's Wort
How To Use: Dilute ½ teaspoon of tinctures made of these herbs in water; consume 2–3 times daily.

Herb: Garlic or Ginger
How To Use: Eat one to two cloves of garlic daily, OR one to two thin ginger slices daily.
Herb: Chamomile
How To Use: Poultice, compress and/or infusion; for infusion — drink and/or use cotton pads to apply it over itchy skin.

#17. Cold (common)
Herb: Ginger
How To Use: Infuse one gram of fresh ginger root with ¾ cup of water for five minutes; drink up to three cups daily.

#18. Cold Sore
Herb: Lemon balm
How To Use: Purchase or make lip balm with 1% lemon balm content, or make an infusion or compress.

#19. Colic
Herb: Ginger
How To Use: For best results, mix ¼ teaspoon ground ginger powder with ¼ cup hot water; drink one to two times daily.
Herb: Slippery elm
How To Use: For best results, use powder; dissolve one teaspoon in one cup of hot water. If it is too thick, you can add more water; sweeten it to taste. (For children and babies, do not exceed ⅛ teaspoon; adults are limited to 50 grams daily).

#20. Colitis
Herb: Aloe vera, Turmeric, or Chamomile
How To Use: Consume eight ounces of aloe vera juice, or NO more than one gram of aloe gel, daily for a short time. (Prolonged use can cause damage); OR make turmeric tea a.k.a "golden milk"; OR a chamomile infusion and drink three cups daily.

#21. Conjunctivitis (pink eye)
Herb: Green tea
How To Use: Steep two green tea bags in hot water for 10 minutes; squeeze out excess liquid; refrigerate tea bags for 20 minutes; place them over your eyelids; let them sit for up to 30 minutes (You can also make a compress with loose leaf tea.)

#22. Constipation
Herb: Dandelion root
How To Use: Decoction made with 20 grams of root and 750 milliliters of water; drink 450–600 milliliters daily.

#23. Cough
Herb: Peppermint
How To Use: Infusion, decoction, or tincture; OR use seven to eight drops of essential oil for steam inhalation as needed.
Herb: Thyme
How To Use: Infuse two teaspoons of crushed leaves in one cup of boiling water; steep for 10 minutes; drink 2–3 times daily.

Herb: Ginger
How To Use: Infuse one-inch fresh ginger root in a cup of hot water for 10–15 minutes; drink up to three cups daily.

#24. Cystitis
Herb: Garlic or Echinacea
How To Use: For best results, use pills or capsules of either herb, 300 milligrams, two to three times daily.

#25. Dandruff
Herb: Aloe vera
How To Use: Apply extracted aloe gel over the scalp; wrap your head in a towel; let it sit for 30 minutes; rinse your scalp with a mild shampoo.

#26. Diaper Rash
Herbs: Aloe vera and/or Calendula
How To Use: Ointment or cream applied to the affected area as needed.
Herb: Lavender
How To Use: Melt ¼ cup of coconut oil; remove from heat and add 10–20 drops of pure lavender essential oil; mix, pour into an airtight container, cool, and store; use as needed.

#27. Diabetes
Herb: Milk thistle
How To Use: Take pills, capsules, or powder supplements daily to reduce insulin resistance (best for Type 2 diabetes).
Herb: Ginger
How To Use: Infuse powdered ginger or fresh ginger slices into hot water, OR take 300-milligram capsules or pills daily.

#28. Diarrhea
Herb: Agrimony and/or Sage
How To Use: Decoction with one tablespoon of either herb; simmer in one cup of water for 15–20 minutes; ONLY drink 450 milliliters daily for three days. (Too much may impair your bowel tissue's ability to absorb nutrients in the food you eat.)

#29. Digestive inflammation (GERD)
Herb: Licorice
How To Use: Take over-the-counter or homemade licorice tablets to alleviate GERD symptoms and protect you from too much acid production.
Herb: Chamomile or Peppermint
How To Use: Make an infusion, decoction, or tincture.
Herb: Slippery elm
How To Use: Take pills, powders, or capsules. Powdered form — mix one tablespoon in tea or water; drink up to three times daily (optional to add honey or sweetener).

#30. Earache
Herb: Garlic
How To Use: Infused oil — put one to two drops on a cotton ball and plug the affected ear, or put one drop directly into the ear and plug with a cotton ball.

#31. Eczema
Herb: Chickweed and/or Nettle
How To Use: Apply creams or ointment to the affected area up to five times daily.
Herb: Peppermint
How To Use: Cream or ointment applied to the affected area 2–3 times daily, OR poultice applied for 20 minutes.
Herbs: Aloe vera
How To Use: Aloe gel applied topically

#32. Fatigue
Herb: Echinacea (Dried)
How To Use: Infuse one teaspoon of herb for every cup of hot water; let steep for five to ten minutes; drink two to four cups daily.
Herb: Peppermint or Rosemary
How To Use: Use steam inhalation with either essential oils with 10–20 drops in a warm bath, vaporizer, or diffuser.

#33. Fever
Herb: Yarrow and Elderberry
How To Use: Infusion with ½ teaspoon of each herb brewed in 100 milliliters of hot water for 10 minutes; drink 600 milliliters daily.

#34. Fractures
Herb: Turmeric
How To Use: Internal use — drink turmeric tea (golden milk); OR external compress application made with turmeric and onion paste.
Herb: Nettle
How To Use: nfuse one cup of dried nettle leaves into one liter of boiling water; then simmer for at least four hours; strain and drink one cup three times daily (cold or warm).

#35. Gastritis
Herb: Garlic
How To Use: Take or make garlic extract supplements, OR eat more garlic regularly.
Herb: Ginger
How To Use: Infuse one part ginger to five parts boiling water; steep for five minutes; drink throughout the day.
Herb: Chamomile
How To Use: Infuse one to two teaspoons of dried chamomile flowers in a cup of hot water; steep for at least five minutes; drink three times daily.

#36. Gingivitis (gum inflammation)
Herb: Sage
How To Use: Make a mouthwash with two tablespoons of fresh sage leaves or one dried leaf; drain, cool, swish in your mouth, then spit; do this 2–3 times daily.
Herb: Aloe vera
How To Use: Pure aloe vera juice purchased at local supermarkets; swish the undiluted juice for 30 seconds and spit; do this two to three times daily.

#37. Hair loss
Herb: Aloe vera or Holy basil
How To Use: Make an ointment, cream, or salve depending on the consistency you desire; with clean hands, apply directly on your scalp; gently massage until the skin absorbs the formula; wash out or leave in.

#38. Halitosis (bad breath)
Herb: Cloves or Parsley
How To Use: Simply sucking on some clove or fresh parsley leaves will temporarily improve halitosis.
Herb: Green tea
How To Use: Infuse one to two cups daily or chew on fresh leaves.

#39. Hangover
Herb: Dandelion (Dried)
How To Use: Decoction made with 15 grams of dandelion root and three cups of water; drink it in small quantities throughout your day.

#40. Headache
Herb: Skullcap (Dried)
How To Use: Infuse and drink no more than three cups daily.
Herb: Peppermint and/or Lavender
How To Use: Use about one teaspoon of carrier oil (coconut, grapeseed, etc.) Massage essential oils into your temples or at the base of your skull along the hairline
Herb: Catnip (Dried)
How To Use: Infuse one to two teaspoons in hot water; brew for 10–15 minutes; drink with honey or lemon to improve its woody taste.

#41. Heartburn (acid reflux)
Herb: Slippery elm
How To Use: Mix two tablespoons of slippery elm bark powder in three tablespoons of COLD water; stir the paste into one cup of BOILING water; add a pinch of cinnamon or nutmeg to improve the taste.
Herb: Ginger
How To Use: Infuse one cup of water with a one-inch chunk of fresh ginger for five minutes; steep for 20 more minutes; strain into a cup; stir and sweeten to taste.

#42. Hemorrhoids
Herb: Slippery elm
How to Use: Pills or capsules taken by mouth, OR drink an infusion made with One tO three teaspoons of powder in hot water three times daily.

#43. High blood pressure
Herb: Garlic
How to Use: Take garlic tablets or eat fresh garlic cloves daily.
Herb: Ginger
How to Use: Eat raw or grated over salad; make infusions; OR take supplements (three to four grams extract daily).

#44. Hives
Herb: Dandelion root
How To Use: Consume a decoction prepared with five grams of root to 750 milliliters of water daily.
Herb: Aloe vera
How To Use: Ointment applied on the area topically as needed.
Herb: Chickweed
How To Use: Cream applied over the affected skin as needed.

#45. Indigestion
Herb: Chamomile
How To Use: Prepare an infusion with one to two teaspoons of chamomile in boiling water for 10 minutes; add honey if preferred.
Herb: Fennel seeds
How To Use: Infuse ½ teaspoon of crushed seeds in one cup of boiling water for 10 minutes, OR simply chew on the seeds.

#46. Insect bites
Herbs: Thyme, Chamomile, and/or Lemon balm; Nettle
How To Use: Make a poultice from one or more of the above herbs; apply it over the insect bite; let it sit for around 10 minutes; OR make a compress or lotion. Internal remedy — nettle infusion three times daily for three days.

#47. Insomnia (sleeplessness)
Herb: Chamomile, Lavender, and/or Passionflower
How To Use: Make an infusion from one or more of the above herbs with one to two heaping teaspoons in 150 milliliters of water; try one or a mixture to find which one works best for you.
Herb: Bergamot, St. John's Wort, and/or Valerian
How To Use: Aromatherapy — either extract the essential oils from these herbs yourself or purchase trusted brands. Use one teaspoon of carrier oil (coconut, grapeseed, etc.) and one drop of essential oil; massage your forehead, neck, wrist, and temples before bed.

#48. Liver infection
Herb: Milk thistle, Turmeric, and/or Garlic
How To Use: Pills, powders, or capsules of any of the above (store-bought or homemade); OR eat two cloves of garlic daily.

#49. Menopause
Herb: Sage
How To Use: Infuse ½ ounce of fresh sage leaves in four cups of water; drink through your day; use as needed.
Herb: St. John's wort
How To Use: Mix ½ teaspoon of tincture with a cup of water; drink up to three times daily.

#50. Mental focus (mental fatigue)
Herb: Gingko
How To Use: Make or purchase pills or capsules; take 120–240 milligrams daily for three months.

#51. Migraine
Herb: Skullcap and/or Rosemary

How To Use: Infusion made with one teaspoon of dried herbs and 3/5 cups of water; choose one or mix them up; ONLY TAKE 600 milliliters per day; also chew on fresh Rosemary stems.

#52. Muscle cramps
Herb: Chamomile
How To Use: Mix one tablespoon of carrier oil (coconut, grapeseed, etc.) with three drops of essential oil and massage directly on the affected muscles.
Herb: Turmeric, Cinnamon, and/or Ginger
How To Use: All these herbs contain curcumin which helps relax muscles. Take a curcumin supplement daily, OR make pills and capsules at home.

#53. Nausea
Herbs: Ginger or Turmeric
How To Use: Take one to two slices of ginger OR up to ½ teaspoon of turmeric and infuse it in 150 milliliters of water for five minutes, as needed.
Herb: Peppermint
How To Use: Headaches with nausea — infuse 150 milliliters of water and one teaspoon of peppermint; drink up to three cups daily.

#54. Period pains
Herb: Lavender, Peppermint, and/or Fennel
How To Use: Mix one tablespoon of carrier oil (coconut, grapeseed, etc.) with three drops of essential oil; massage directly on the affected area.

#55. Premenstrual syndrome (PMS)
Herb: Valerian
How To Use: Take pills or capsules purchased or homemade, OR 20–40 drops of tincture in water drank up to five times daily.
Herb: Rosemary
How To Use: External application — Infuse one tablespoon of dried leaves or two tablespoons of fresh leaves in a liter of water; strain the infusion into a warm bath in the morning; soak for 20 minutes.

#56. Psoriasis
Herb: Aloe vera and/or Turmeric
How To Use: Purchase or make aloe vera cream with at least 0.5% aloe; apply to the affected skin up to three times daily for five days; take two days off, then reapply. After a maximum of four weeks, let your skin breathe by taking a break for a few weeks.
Herb: Turmeric
How To Use: Cream, ointment, compress, or poultice made from fresh minced or powdered root; apply to the affected area three times a day for no more than four weeks.

#57. Rheumatoid arthritis
Herb: Green tea
How To Use: Drink hot or cold infusions three to four times daily.
Herb: Cinnamon
How To Use: Add an extra sprinkle of cinnamon over your dishes or to your infusions.

#58. Shingles
Herb: Lemon balm
How To Use: Drink infusions daily, OR make and/or purchase supplements.
Herb: Chamomile
How To Use: Mix one tablespoon of carrier oil (coconut, grapeseed, etc.) with three drops of essential oil; massage directly on the affected area.

#59. Sinus infection
Herb: Garlic and/or Ginger
How To Use: Add a few teaspoons of fresh garlic or ginger to your meals; OR, drink ginger infusions three times daily.

#60. Skin tags
Herb: Garlic
How To Use: Apply crushed garlic over the affected area; cover it with a clean cloth or bandage and let it sit overnight; wash the area thoroughly in the morning; repeat as needed.
Herb: Ginger
How To Use: Clean the skin first and pat dry; take slices of fresh ginger and gently rub over the skin tag for one minute; repeat as needed.

#61. Sore throat
Herb: Rosemary, Sage, Myrrh, and Echinacea
How To Use: Dissolve one teaspoon of EACH herbs' tincture in five teaspoons of warm water; gargle and swallow (DO NOT swallow if pregnant).
Herb: Licorice root
How To Use: Steep one tablespoon of minced root in one cup of hot water for five minutes, strain, and add honey if desired.
Herb: Ginger
How To Use: Infuse one tablespoon of ginger in one cup of hot water; cover and steep for 10 minutes; add a sweetener of choice; enjoy hot or cold.

#62. Sprains
Herb: Turmeric and/or Garlic
How To Use: Poultice made with one or both herbs; apply on the sprained area; wrap a clean bandage to secure in place for a few hours; repeat as needed.
Herb: Arnica or Comfrey
How To Use: Cream, ointment, or infused oil applied to the affected area three times daily (DO NOT use on broken skin).

#63. Stiff joints
Herb: St. John's Wort or Comfrey and Lavender
How To Use: Mix 2 ½ tablespoons of either St. John's wort OR comfrey infused oil with 20–40 drops of lavender essential oil, then massage remedy over the area of concern.

#64. Stomach spasms
Herb: LemOn balm and Angelica
How To Use: Infuse three parts lemon balm and one part angelica in hot water; drink a maximum of 750 milliliters daily.

Herb: Peppermint
How To Use: Make infusions, chew on fresh leaves, or suck on organic peppermint candy.
Herb: Ginger
How To Use: Purchase or make ginger supplements; OR drink infusions or non-alcoholic ginger beer (a.k.a. ginger ale).

#65. Stones (bladder, gall, and kidney)
Herb: Asparagus
How To Use: Add more asparagus to your diet.
Herb: Dandelion and Parsley
How To Use: Infuse two cups of fresh chopped parsley in six cups of boiling water for five minutes; remove from heat; steep for 10 minutes; strain and add four teaspoons of dandelion root powder; drink the entire six cups before bed; repeat every night for one to two weeks. (May dissolve or the pass stone, which may be painful).

#66. Stress
Herbs: Lavender, Valerian, Passionflower, and Ginger
How To Use: Combine six teaspoons dried lavender, one teaspoon dried valerian root, ½ teaspoon dried ginger with one teaspoon dried orange peels, and 180 milliliters alcohol to make a tincture; take one dropper full as needed.

#67. Sunburn
Herbs: Aloe vera; Lavender
How To Use: Apply aloe vera gel; OR mix one tablespoon of carrier oil (coconut, grapeseed, etc.) with three drops of essential oil; apply to affected areas.

#68. Swelling and fluid retention
Herb: Dandelion, Hawthorn, OR Green tea
How To Use: Take these herbs as infusions or decoctions as needed.

#69. Tongue ulcers
Herb: Myrrh, Echinacea, and Licorice
How To Use: Mix equal parts of each herbal tincture; apply to the affected area in the mouth; do this every hour.

#70. Tonsillitis
Herb: Echinacea
How To Use: Gargle with echinacea decoctions as needed.
Herb: Cinnamon
How To Use: In a cup of hot water, add one teaspoon of cinnamon powder; add honey if desired; sip while warm two to three times daily.
Herb: Turmeric
How To Use: Mix ½ teaspoon of turmeric powder and ½ teaspoon of salt in warm water and gargle; use once in the morning and again at night.

#71. Travel sickness
Herb: Lavender, Peppermint, or Ginger
How To Use: Inhale essential oils, OR apply infused oil under the nose and on temples.

#72. Urinary tract infection (UTI)
Herb: Garlic or Echinacea
How To Use: Purchase or make capsules or tablets
(MAY ALSO USE #65–STONE REMEDIES)

#73. Varicose veins
Herb: Yarrow
How to Use: Wash affected areas with a cool yarrow infusion, OR apply ointment or cream.

#74. Vertigo (dizzy spells)
Herb: Ginger
How To Use: Drink infusion by steeping either freshly peeled ginger root or prepared ginger tea bags.
Herb: Lavender; Peppermint; Ginger
How To Use: Three to five drops of any of these essential oils in a diffuser; OR mix one tablespoon of carrier oil (coconut, grapeseed, etc.) with three drops of essential oil; apply to temples and base of the neck.

#75. Warts
Herb: Aloe vera
How To Use: Rub aloe vera gel over the wart 2–3 times daily for three months.
Herb: Garlic
How To Use: Crush one to two cloves in water; apply over the affected areas; cover with a clean cloth; let sit for 10–20 minutes; repeat daily for three months.

#76. Wounds
Herb: Yarrow or St. John's Wort
How To Use: Tincture or poultice; OR infused oil, ointments, and/or creams applied topically.
Herb: Comfrey
How To Use: Use an ointment around the edges of your wound. A poultice is recommended for injuries that already have scab formation.

#77. Yeast infection
Herb: Oregano
How To Use: Mix three drops of essential oil with two tablespoons of olive oil, coconut oil, or almond oil; apply internally into the vagina at night before bed. You may also purchase oregano oil capsules.
Herb: Comfrey
How To Use: Poultice can be applied to the affected area and held in place with a clean bandage or cloth; leave on for one to two hours daily.

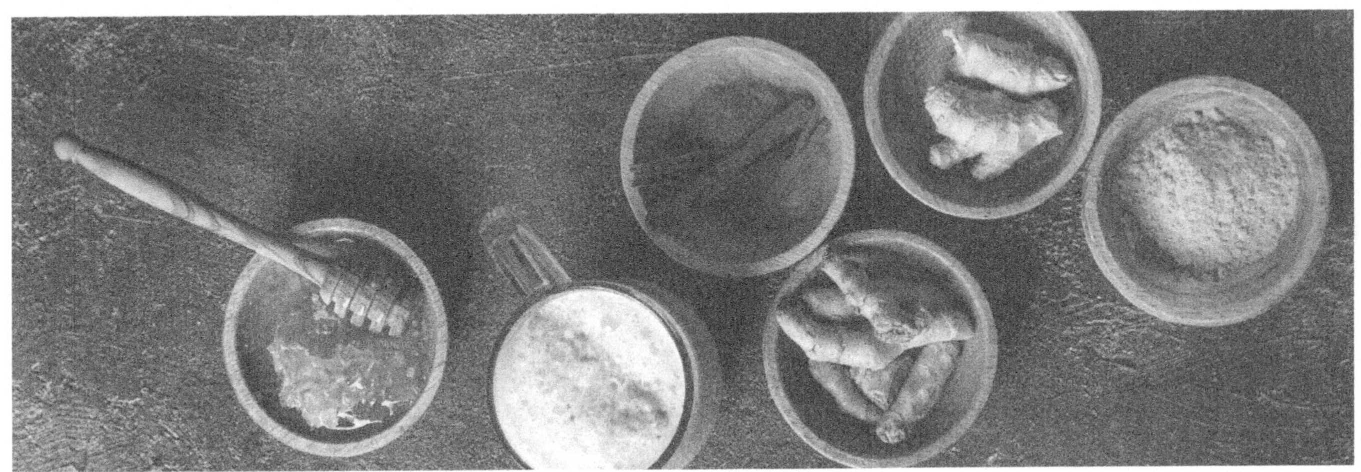

Bonus Recipe

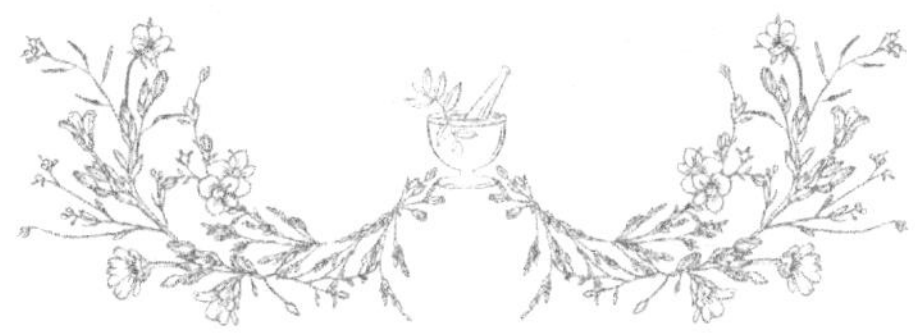

Vital Golden Milk

Things you will need:

- 1 cup unsweetened milk or milk alternative
- 1 teaspoon honey (up to 1 tablespoon or more, to taste)
- ¼ teaspoon ground turmeric
- ¼ teaspoon ground ginger (can sub 1-2 teaspoons fresh grated ginger, to taste)
- 1 - 5-inch cinnamon stick (can sub ⅛ teaspoon ground cinnamon)
- Pinch of black pepper (enhances the anti-inflammatory effects of turmeric)
- ½ teaspoon pure organic vanilla extract
- ½ teaspoon coconut oil (optional)

Preparation:

1.) Set a small saucepan over LOW heat, Then add everything BUT the vanilla and coconut oil (if using).

2.) STEAM, just below a simmer. DO NOT let it come to a boil! Keep just simmering, occasionally stirring, for 10 minutes.

3.) Stir in the vanilla and coconut oil (optional). Taste and add additional honey if desired. (I like about two teaspoons.)

4.) If desired, you can use a frother to froth the tea. Pour into a mug and spoon the foam over the top. ENJOY!

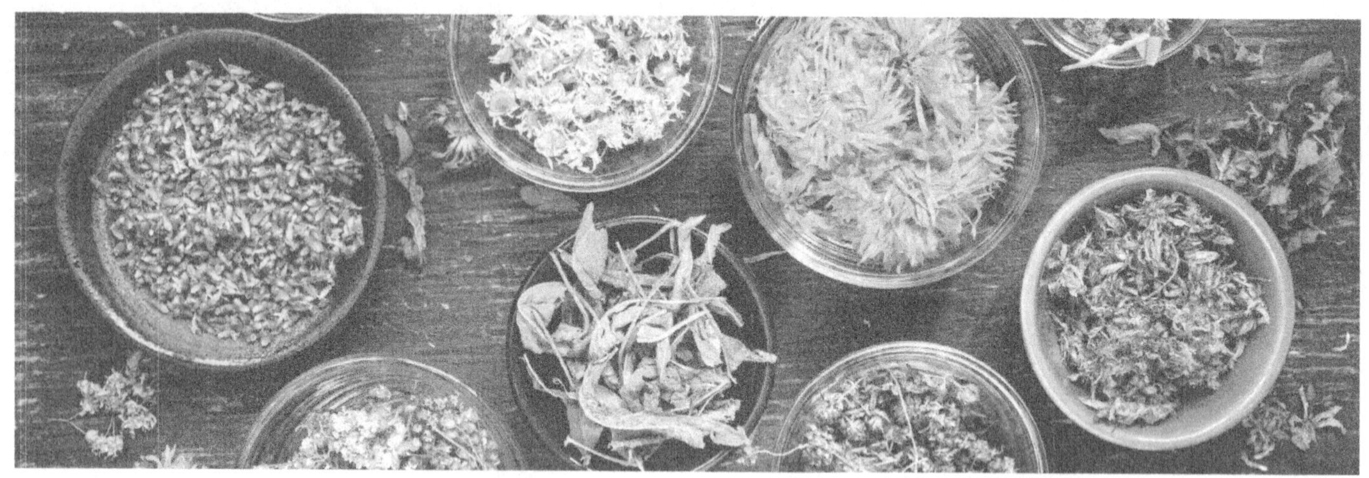

Conclusion

Please give yourself a pat on the back and a well-deserved congratulations for making it to the end! You now have the tools to embark into the wonders of herbalism and understand fully how medicinal herbs and plants can aid you in all areas of your life. You must remain vigilant to ensure that your body maintains its utmost healthy state.

After exploring the rich history of herbalism, you absorbed the fundamentals, dug deeper into the five pillars of optimal health and vitality, and got acquainted with 54 amazing herbs to get you started toward your holistic goals. THEN, you discovered 17 herbal preparation techniques and many ways to begin implementing them in your life.

With simple tools and your knowledge of herbs, preparing them to fit your needs is something you can master with practice and research. Nourish your expertise in growing different herbs, preparing them, and knowing when and where they are beneficial! After becoming confident about your skills in your newfound lifestyle, you can help your friends and family live holistically by educating them about the immense benefits they can get from herbalism.

Hopefully, this book has enlightened you on what your journey in herbalism will be like soon. Herbalism is a lifestyle that involves careful research, a keen eye for identifying herbs, and lots of patience to help you remain consistent in learning more each day.

On Small Request...

As a self published auther, reviews are an enormous help! **It would mean the world to me** if you could leave a review. If you enjoyed reading this book and learned a thing or two... **please leave an Amazon review. It takes less than 30 seconds but means so much to me!**

Thank you and I can not wait to read your thoughts.

Have questions or need support on your herbal journey?

Come Join Our Herbal Family!

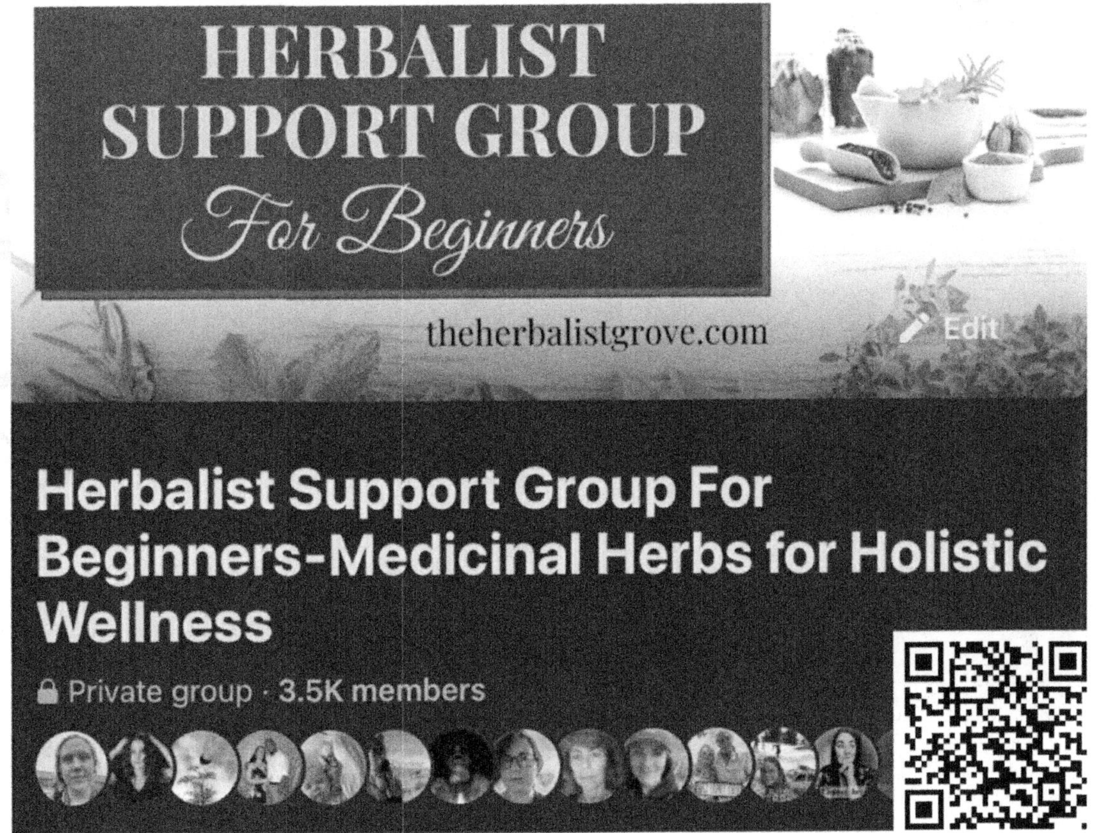

Connect with like-minded individuals in our private Facebook community!

GO TO Theherbalistgrove.com or

SCAN the QR code above to

JOIN NOW!

Index

77 Common Ailments Index

Resources

CHAPTER 1

Atanasov, A. G., Waltenberger, B., Pferschy-Wenzig, E.-M., Linder, T., Wawrosch, C., Uhrin, P., Temml, V., Wang, L., Stuppner, H., Dirsch, V. M., Bauer, R., Kopp, B., Mihovilovic, M. D., Bochkov, V., Breuss, J. M., Schuster, D., Rollinger, J. M., Heiss, E. H., & Schwaiger, S. (2015). Discovery and resupply of pharmacologically active plant-derived natural products: A Review. *Draw Science, 33*(8), 1582–1614. https://doi.org/10.18516/0001

Cartwright, M. (2021, June 9). *The Spice Trade & The Age of Exploration.* World History Encyclopedia. https://www.worldhistory.org/article/1777/the-spice-trade--the-age-of-exploration/

Dafni, A., & Böck, B. (2019). Medicinal plants of the Bible—revisited. *Journal of Ethnobiology and Ethnomedicine, 15*(1). https://doi.org/10.1186/s13002-019-0338-8

Hajar, R. (2012). The air of history (part II) medicine in the Middle Ages. *Heart Views, 13*(4), 158. https://doi.org/10.4103/1995-705x.105744

Hassan, H. M. (2015). A short history of the use of plants as medicines from ancient times. *CHIMIA International Journal for Chemistry, 69*(10), 622–623. https://doi.org/10.2533/chimia.2015.622

Petrovska, B. B. (2012). Historical review of medicinal plants' usage. *Pharmacognosy Reviews, 6*(11), 1. https://doi.org/10.4103/0973-7847.95849

Ravishankar, B., & Shukla, V. J. (2008). Indian systems of Medicine: A Brief Profile. *African Journal of Traditional, Complementary and Alternative Medicines, 4*(3), 319. https://doi.org/10.4314/ajtcam.v4i3.31226

Sallam, H. N. (2010). Aristotle, Godfather of Evidence-Based Medicine. *Facts, Views & Vision in ObGyn, 2*(1), 11–19.

Scott Nokes, R. (2004). The several compilers of Bald's leechbook. *Anglo-Saxon England, 33*, 51–76. https://doi.org/10.1017/s0263675104000031

Sellami, M., Slimeni, O., Pokrywka, A., Kuvačić, G., D Hayes, L., Milic, M., & Padulo, J. (2018). *Herbal Medicine for Sports: A Review. Journal of the International Society of Sports Nutrition, 15*(1). https://doi.org/10.1186/s12970-018-0218-y

Worth Estes, J. (1995). The European Reception of the First Drugs from the New World. *Pharmacy in History, 37(*1), 3–23. https://doi.org/https://www.jstor.org/stable/41111660

Zeisel, S. H. (1999). Regulation of "nutraceuticals". *Science, 285*(5435), 1853–1855. https://doi.org/10.1126/science.285.5435.1853

CHAPTER 2

A glossary of herbal medicine terms. The Upside by Vitacost.com. (2020, January 14). https://www.vitacost.com/blog/herbal-medicine-glossary/

Terminology. Terminology Page - American Botanical Council. (n.d.). https://www.herbalgram.org/resources/terminology-page/

The herbalist's vocabulary cheat sheet. Herbal Academy. (2017, September 17). https://theherbalacademy.com/herbalists-vocabulary-cheat-sheet/

CHAPTER 3

American Botanical Council (ABC). (n.d.) Terminology. https://www.herbalgram.org/resources/terminology-page/

Benzie, I. F., & Wachtel-Galor, S. (2011). *Herbal medicine: Biomolecular and clinical aspects.* Boca Raton: CRC Press.

Boyers, L. (2021). What exactly are tannins in tea? Here's everything you need to know. https://www.mindbodygreen.com/articles/tannins-in-tea

Chertoff, J. (2019). What is astringent? https://www.healthline.com/health/beauty-skin-care/astringent

Cronkleton, E. (2020). 8 Natural Sleep Aids: What Works. https://www.healthline.com/health/healthy-sleep/natural-sleep-aids

Dai, J., & Mumper, R. J. (2010). Plant phenolics: extraction, analysis and their antioxidant and anticancer properties. *Molecules (Basel, Switzerland), 15*(10), 7313–7352. https://doi:10.3390/molecules15107313

Desai, Sapna & Desai, D.G. & Kaur, Harmeet. (2009). Saponins and their biological activities. Pharma Times. 41. 13-16.

Evans, S. (2008). Changing the knowledge base in Western herbal medicine. *Social Science & Medicine, 67*(12), 2098-2106. https://doi:10.1016/j.socscimed.2008.09.046

Hartmann, T. (2007). From waste products to ecochemicals: Fifty years research of plant secondary metabolism. *Phytochemistry, 68*(22-24), 2831-2846. https://doi:10.1016/j.phytochem.2007.09.017

Hillsborough Homesteading. (2020). Top 18 herbal actions and how to use them. https://hillsborough-homesteading.com/top-herbal-actions-how-to-use/

Hussain, G., Rasul, A., Anwar, H., Aziz, N., Razzaq, A., Wei, W., Ali, M., Li, J., & Li, X. (2018). Role of Plant Derived Alkaloids and Their Mechanism in Neurodegenerative Disorders. *International journal of biological sciences, 14*(3), 341–357. https://doi.org/10.7150/ijbs.23247

Lehman, S. (2021). Health benefits of vegetables with glucosinolates. https://www.verywellfit.com/what-are-glucosinolates-and-why-are-they-good-for-me-2505908

Li, J. W., & Vederas, J. (2011). Drug discovery and natural products: End of era or an endless frontier? *Biomeditsinskaya Khimiya, 57*(2), 148-160. http://doi:10.18097/pbmc20115702148

Marglin, E. (2021). A glossary of herbal medicine terms. https://www.vitacost.com/blog/herbal-medicine-glossary/

Martínez-Pérez, E. F., Juárez, Z. N., Hernández, L. R., & Bach, H. (2018). Natural Antispasmodics: Source, Stereochemical Configuration, and Biological Activity. *BioMed research international, 2018*, 3819714. https://doi.org/10.1155/2018/3819714

McDermott, A. (2018). 5 Herbal Remedies for Constipation. https://www.healthline.com/health/digestive-health/herbal-remedies-for-constipation

Mishra, S., Pandey, A., & Manvati, S. (2020). *Coumarin: An emerging antiviral agent. Heliyon, 6(1), e03217.* http://doi:10.1016/j.heliyon.2020.e03217

Seeff, L., Stickel, F., & Navarro, V. J. (2013). Hepatotoxicity of Herbals and Dietary Supplements. *Drug-Induced Liver Disease,* 631-657. http://doi:10.1016/b978-0-12-387817-5.00035-2

Shamsi-Baghbanan, H., Sharifian, A., Esmaeili, S., & Minaei, B. (2014). Hepatoprotective herbs, avicenna viewpoint. *Iranian Red Crescent medical journal, 16*(1), e12313. http://doi:10.5812/ircmj.12313

Stefanachi, A., Leonetti, F., Pisani, L., Catto, M., & Carotti, A. (2018). Coumarin: A Natural, Privileged and Versatile Scaffold for Bioactive Compounds. *Molecules (Basel, Switzerland), 23*(2), 250. http://doi:10.3390/molecules23020250

Tilburt, J. (2008). Herbal medicine research and global health: An ethical analysis. *Bulletin of the World Health Organization, 86*(8), 594-599. http://doi:10.2471/blt.07.042820

United States Department of Agriculture (USDA). (n.d.). Active plant ingredients used for medicinal purposes. https://www.fs.fed.us/wildflowers/ethnobotany/medicinal/ingredients.shtml

Watson, K. (2019). What are flavonoids? Everything you need to know. https://www.healthline.com/health/what-are-flavonoids-everything-you-need-to-know

Weiss, R. F. (2001). What is Herbal Medicine? In *Weiss's Herbal Medicine* (Classic ed., pp. 1–2). Thieme.

CHAPTER 4

Carpenter, S. (2001, October). *Sleep deprivation may be undermining teen health.* Monitor on Psychology. http://www.apa.org/monitor/oct01/sleepteen

Cortisol. You and your hormones. (2019, January). https://www.yourhormones.info/hormones/cortisol/

Dulloo, A. G., Duret, C., Rohrer, D., Girardier, L., Mensi, N., Fathi, M., Chantre, P., & Vandermander, J. (1999). Efficacy of a green tea extract rich in catechin polyphenols and caffeine in increasing 24-H energy expenditure and fat oxidation in humans. *The American Journal of Clinical Nutrition, 70*(6), 1040–1045. https://doi.org/10.1093/ajcn/70.6.1040

Foster, S. (1995, June). Herbs for health: *A good night's sleep.* Mother Earth Living. https://content.motherearthliving.com/health-and-wellness/herbs-for-health-a-good-nights-sleep/

Klein, S. (2013, April 19). *The 3 major stress hormones, explained.* HuffPost. http://www.huffpost.com/entry/adrenaline-cortisol-stress-hormones_n_3112800

Krishnamurti, C., & amp; Rao, S. S. C. C. (2016). The isolation of morphine by Serturner. *Indian Journal of Anaesthesia, 60*(11), 861. https://doi.org/10.4103/0019-5049.193696

Kubala, J. (2018, June 12). *Essential amino acids: Definition, benefits and food sources.* Healthline. http://www.healthline.com/nutrition/essential-amino-acids

Micronutrients: Vitamins and minerals. Fit for performance weight loss strategies . (n.d.). https://phc.amedd.army.mil/PHC%20Resource%20Library/FFP-4-MicronutrientsVitaminsandMinerals.pdf

Park, H. R., Park, M., Choi, J., Park, K.-Y., Chung, H. Y., & Lee, J. (2010). A high-fat diet impairs neurogenesis: Involvement of lipid peroxidation and brain-derived neurotrophic factor. *Neuroscience Letters, 482*(3), 235–239. https://doi.org/10.1016/j.neulet.2010.07.046

Peri, C. (2014). 10 Things to Hate About Sleep Loss. https://www.webmd.com/sleep-disorders/features/10-results-sleep-loss

Rautio, S. (2018, September 25). *Increase intake of fresh herbs for everyday health. MSU Extension.* http://www.canr.msu.edu/news/increase_intake_of_fresh_herbs_for_everyday_health

Roberts, D. D. H. (2020, July 6). *Understanding the stress response.* Harvard Health. http://www.health.harvard.edu/staying-healthy/understanding-the-stress-response

Srivastava, J. K., Shankar, E., & Gupta, S. (2010). Chamomile: A herbal medicine of the past with a bright future. *Molecular medicine reports, 3*(6), 895–

901. https://doi.org/10.3892/mmr.2010.377

U.S. National Library of Medicine. (2020, August 18). *BDNF gene: Medlineplus genetics.* MedlinePlus. http://www.medlineplus.gov/genetics/gene/bdnf/

What foods have a thermogenic effect? 17 foods with thermogenic effect. GrowBigZen. (2021, May 6). http://www.growbigzen.com/what-foods-have-a-thermogenic-effect-17-foods-with-thermogenic-effect/

Chapter 5

American Botanical Council (ABC). (n.d.) Skullcap. https://www.herbalgram.org/resources/herbalgram/issues/83/table-of-contents/herbalgram-83-herb-profile-skullcap/

Arnica Montana L. (n.d.). https://www.avogel.com/plant-encyclopaedia/arnica_montana.php

Ashpari, Z. (2018, September 29). The calming effects of passionflower. https://www.healthline.com/health/anxiety/calming-effects-of-passionflower

Augustyn, A., Zeidan, A., Zelazko, A., Eldridge, A., McKenna, A., Tikkanen, A., ... World Data Editors (Eds.). (2021, September 21). hemp. Encyclopædia Britannica. https://www.britannica.com/plant/hemp

Benzie, I. F., & Wachtel-Galor, S. (2011). *Herbal medicine: Biomolecular and clinical aspects.* Boca Raton: CRC Press.

Britannica. (n.d.). Bay leaf. https://www.britannica.com/topic/bay-leaf

Butler, N. (2019, April 01). Can hops help you sleep? https://www.healthline.com/health/can-hops-get-me-to-sleep

Cafasso, J. (2019, March 08). The therapeutic capabilities of slippery elm bark. https://www.healthline.com/health/food-nutrition/slippery-elm-bark

Cannalisteu. (2021, June 1). 12 benefits of hemp seed oil for Great Health. CannaList EU. https://www.cannalist.eu/12-benefits-of-hemp-seed-oil-for-great-health/amp/

Chacko, S. M., Thambi, P. T., Kuttan, R., & Nishigaki, I. (2010). Beneficial effects of green tea: a literature review. *Chinese medicine, 5*, 13. https://doi.org/10.1186/1749-8546-5-13

Chevallier, A. (2016). Encyclopedia of Herbal Medicine (3rd ed.). DK Publishing.

Cinnamon cultivation and processing in India. Kisan Suvidha. (2017, October 26). http://www.kisansuvidha.com/cinnamon/?v=ad4f1670f142

Contributors, W. M. D. E. (2020, December 22). Hemp Seed Oil: Health benefits, nutrition, dosage, and more. WebMD. https://www.webmd.com/diet/health-benefits-hemp-seed-oil#2-5

Cronkleton, E. (2019, March 08). 10 benefits of lemon balm and how to use it. https://www.healthline.com/health/lemon-balm-uses

Cronkleton, E. (2021, September 29). What are the risks and benefits of catnip tea? https://www.medicalnewstoday.com/articles/catnip-tea

Drugs.com. (n.d.) Catnip. https://www.drugs.com/npc/catnip.html

Encyclopedia.com. (2018, May 11). Cayenne. *Gale encyclopedia of alternative medicine.* https://www.encyclopedia.com/places/latin-america-and-caribbean/south-american-political-geography/cayenne

Fanous, S. (2018, September 17). 9 health benefits of thyme. https://www.healthline.com/health/health-benefits-of-thyme

Fanous, S. (2021). 5 possible uses for the bay leaf. https://www.healthline.com/health/5-possible-uses-for-bay-leaf

Fidler, M (2017). History and benefits of eleuthero. https://www.integrativepro.com/articles/history-and-benefits-of-eleuthero

Filippone, P. T. (2019, August 19). *Interesting highlights in the colorful history of cinnamon.* The Spruce Eats. http://www.thespruceeats.com/history-of-cinnamon-1807584

Fobar, R. (2019, December 13). Frankincense trees – of biblical lore – are being tapped out for essential oils. https://www.nationalgeographic.com/animals/article/frankincense-trees-declining-overtapping

Gaia Herbs Farm. (2017, November 13). *Thyme.* Gaia Herbs.
https://www.gaiaherbs.com/blogs/herbs/thyme

Grant, A. (2021). Cayenne pepper in the garden – tips for growing cayenne peppers. https://www.gardeningknowhow.com/edible/vegetables/pepper/growing-cayenne-peppers.htm

Huizen, J. (2017, August 23). 12 potential health benefits of eleuthero. https://www.medicalnewstoday.com/articles/319084#_noHeaderPrefixedContent

Iqbal, M., Bibi, Y., Raja, N. I., Ejaz, M., Hussain, M., Yasmeen, F., . . . Imran, M. (2017). Review on Therapeutic and Pharmaceutically Important Medicinal Plant Asparagus officinalis L. *Journal of Plant Biochemistry & Physiology, 05*(01). https://doi:10.4172/2329-9029.1000180\

James, T. (2016). How to spot wild catnip. https://www.adventurecats.org/pawsome-reads/foraging-adventure-how-to-spot-wild-catnip/

Jamshidi, N., & Cohen, M. M. (2017). The Clinical Efficacy and Safety of Tulsi in Humans: A Systematic Review of the Literature. *Evidence-Based*

Complementary and Alternative Medicine, 2017, 1-13. https://doi:10.1155/2017/9217567

Johnson, J. (2019, February 14). Hemp oil benefit list. https://www.medicalnewstoday.com/articles/324450

Koetter, U. Biendl, M. (n.d.). Hops (Humulus lupulus): A review of its historic and medicinal uses. https://www.herbalgram.org/resources/herbalgram/issues/87/table-of-contents/article3559/

Krans, B. (2020, November 03). The health benefits of holy basil. https://www.healthline.com/health/food-nutrition/basil-benefits

Levenberg, C. (2020). 15 uses and benefits of frankincense essential oil and side effects. https://ilavahemp.com/frankincense-essential-oil/

LiverTox: Clinical and Research Information on Drug-Induced Liver Injury [Internet]. Bethesda (MD): National Institute of Diabetes and Digestive and Kidney Diseases; 2012-. Skullcap. [Updated 2020 Mar 28]. https://www.ncbi.nlm.nih.gov/books/NBK548757/

McCulloch, M. (2018). 14 benefits and uses of rosemary essential oil. https://www.healthline.com/nutrition/rosemary-oil-benefits

Missouri Botanical Garden (MBC). (n.d.). Melissa officianalis. https://www.missouribotanicalgarden.org/PlantFinder/PlantFinderDetails.aspx?kempercode=c857

Nordqvst, J. (2019, March 04). What are the health benefits and risks of lavender? https://www.medicalnewstoday.com/articles/265922

Pegiou, E., Mumm, R., Acharya, P., de Vos, R., & Hall, R. D. (2019). Green and White Asparagus *(Asparagus officinalis)*: A Source of Developmental, Chemical and Urinary Intrigue. *Metabolites*, *10*(1), 17. https://doi.org/10.3390/metabo10010017

Perry, N. (2019, December 17) A love letter to lavender. https://www.healthline.com/health/lavender-history-plant-care-types

Petre, A. (2021, March 08). 5 benefits and uses of frankincense – and 7 myths. https://www.healthline.com/nutrition/frankincense

Raman, R. (2017, March 18). 8 impressive health benefits of cayenne pepper. https://www.healthline.com/nutrition/8-benefits-of-cayenne-pepper

Redland Daily Facts (RDF). (2015, November 23). Parsley: A popular herb with a long history. https://www.redlandsdailyfacts.com/2015/11/23/parsley-a-popular-herb-with-a-long-history/

Rodriguez-Leyva, D., & Pierce, G. N. (2010). The cardiac and haemostatic effects of dietary hempseed. *Nutrition & metabolism*, *7*, 32. https://doi.org/10.1186/1743-7075-7-32

Rowles, A. (2020, July 07). 9 benefits and uses of oregano oil. https://www.healthline.com/nutrition/9-oregano-oil-benefits-and-uses

Selles, S., Kouidri, M., Belhamiti, B. T., & Ait Amrane, A. (2020). Chemical composition, in-vitro antibacterial and antioxidant activities of *Syzygium aromaticum* essential oil. *Journal of Food Measurement and Characterization*, 1–7. Advance online publication. https://doi.org/10.1007/s11694-020-00482-5

Semeco, A. (2018, February 28). 7 health benefits of ginseng. https://www.healthline.com/nutrition/ginseng-benefits#TOC_TITLE_HDR_1

Singh, J., Baghotia, A., & Goel, SP. (2012). Eugenia caryophyllata Thunberg (Family Myrtaceae): A Review. International Journal of Research in Pharmaceutical and Biomedical Sciences. 3. 1469-1475. https://www.researchgate.net/profile/Jitender-Singh-4/publication/310799727_Eugenia_caryophyllata_Thunberg_Family_Myrtaceae_A_Review

Singletary, K. (2010). Oregano. *Nutrition Today, 45*(3), 129-138. https://doi:10.1097/nt.0b013e3181dec789

Spices Board India. (n.d.) Bay leaf. http://www.indianspices.com/spice-catalog/bay-leaf.html

Spritzler, F. (2017, April 16). How valerian root help you relax and sleep better. https://www.healthline.com/nutrition/valerian-root

Srivastava, J. K., Shankar, E., & Gupta, S. (2010). Chamomile: A herbal medicine of the past with a bright future. *Molecular medicine reports*, *3*(6), 895–901. https://doi.org/10.3892/mmr.2010.377

Stevinson, C., Devaraj, V. S., Fountain-Barber, A., Hawkins, S., & Ernst, E. (2003). Homeopathic arnica for prevention of pain and bruising: randomized placebo-controlled trial in hand surgery. *Journal of the Royal Society of Medicine*, *96*(2), 60–65. https://doi.org/10.1258/jrsm.96.2.60

Stinson, A. (2018, November 23). Benefits of passionflower for anxiety and insomnia. https://www.medicalnewstoday.com/articles/323795

Undlin, S. (2020, September 25). *The history of thyme (plus uses of thyme)*. Plantsnap. https://www.plantsnap.com/blog/the-history-of-thyme-plus-uses-of-thyme/

Ware, M. (2021, May 18). What are the health benefits of green tea? https://www.medicalnewstoday.com/articles/269538

Warwick, K. (2021, May 10). 10 proven health benefits of turmeric and curcumin. https://www.healthline.com/nutrition/top-10-evidence-based-health-benefits-of-turmeric

Wong, C. (2021a). What is arnica? https://www.verywellhealth.com/the-benefits-of-arnica-89542

Wong, C. (2021b). What is asparagus extract? https://www.verywellhealth.com/the-benefits-of-asparagus-extract-88610

Wong, C. (2021c). What is chamomile? https://www.verywellhealth.com/the-benefits-of-chamomile-89436

Zammarripa, M. (2019, April 05). 8 impressive health benefits and uses of parsley. https://www.healthline.com/nutrition/parsley-benefits

Chapter 6

Angelica. Our Herb Garden. (2013, May 23). http://www.ourherbgarden.com/herb-history/angelica.html

Atalayabio. (n.d.). https://www.atalayabio.com/en/the-history-of-aloe-vera/

Bantillan, C. (2019, December 12). 5 Emerging Benefits and Uses of Yarrow Tea. https://www.healthline.com/nutrition/yarrow-tea#3.-May-help-reduce-symptoms-of-depression-and-anxiety

Burgess, L. (2017, December 20). 10 potential health benefits of milk thistle. https://www.medicalnewstoday.com/articles/320362#what-is-milk-thistle

Brobst, J. B. (2013). *The Herb Society of America Guide to elderberry part 1*. https://www.herbsociety.org/file_download/inline/a54e481a-e368-4414-af68-2e3d42bc0bec

Caron, M. (2021, February 02). Dandelion Tea Benefits: 15 Shocking Scientific Reasons To Love It. https://www.myteadrop.com/blogs/news/dandelion-tea-benefits

Catherine, Matt, Amy, Snij, Fernley, S., Gareth, . . . Sarah. (2021, September 03). How to grow garlic: A step-by-step guide. https://growingfamily.co.uk/garden-tips/grow-garlic/

Crataegus oxycantha (hawthorn) monograph. Alternative Medicine Review. (2010). https://altmedrev.com/wp-content/uploads/2019/02/v15-2-164.pdf

Dahmer, S., & Scott, E. (2015, February 15). Health Effects of Hawthorn. *Complementary and Alternative Medicine, 81*(4).

Dellwo, A. (2021, November 11). What Is Yarrow? https://www.verywellhealth.com/yarrow-health-benefits-4586386

Encyclopedia.com. (2018, May 21). Goldenseal. *Gale encyclopedia of alternative medicine*. https://www.encyclopedia.com/history/united-states-and-canada/us-history-biographies/goldenseal

Encyclopedia.com. (2018, June 8). Milk thistle. *Gale encyclopedia of alternative medicine*. https://www.encyclopedia.com/places/africa/tunisia-political-geography/milk-thistle

Encyclopedia.com. (2018, June 27). Myrrh. *Gale encyclopedia of alternative medicine*. https://www.encyclopedia.com/plants-and-animals/plants/plants/myrrh

Engels, G. E., & Brinckmann, J. B. (2021). Hawthorn - American Botanical Council. https://www.herbalgram.org/resources/herbalgram/issues/96/table-of-contents/herbalgram-96-herb-profile-hawthorn/

Fischer, F. (2020, September 03). History of Calendula. https://www.gardenguides.com/78027-history-calendula.html

Freed, D. M. F. (2017, June 20). *Hawthorn: Heart healing from physical to spiritual*. Traditional Roots Institute. https://traditionalroots.org/hawthorn-heart-healing-from-physical-to-spiritual/

Gaia Herb Farm. (2021). *An essential guide to nettle: History, benefits & uses*. Gaia Herbs. https://www.gaiaherbs.com/blogs/seeds-of-knowledge/an-essential-guide-to-nettle-history-benefits-and-uses

Goncagul, G., & Ayaz, E. (2010). Antimicrobial Effect of Garlic (Allium sativum) and Traditional Medicine. *Journal of Animal and Veterinary Advances, 9*(1), 1-4. https://doi:10.3923/javaa.2010.1.4

Gunnars, K. (2018, June 28). 11 Proven Health Benefits of Quinoa. https://www.healthline.com/nutrition/11-proven-benefits-of-quinoa#TOC_TITLE_HDR_1

Hill, A. (2018, May 29). 12 Benefits of Ginkgo Biloba (Plus Side Effects & Dosage). https://www.healthline.com/nutrition/ginkgo-biloba-benefits

Howdle, J. (2020, March 22). *Beautiful botanicals - angelica*. Dunnet Bay Distillers. https://www.dunnetbaydistillers.co.uk/news/caithness-life/beautiful-botanicals-angelica/

Hunter, C. (2010, June 20). *Chickweed history, folklore, myth and Magic*. The Practical Herbalist. https://thepracticalherbalist.com/advanced-herbalism/chickweed-myth-and-magic/

Kubala, J. (2019, September 27). 10 Science-Based Benefits of Fennel and Fennel Seeds. https://www.healthline.com/nutrition/fennel-and-fennel-seed-benefits#5.-May-have-cancer-fighting-properties

Lang, A. (2020, April 08). 7 Emerging Uses of Calendula Tea and Extract. https://www.healthline.com/nutrition/calendula-tea

Maruca, G., Laghetti, G., Mafrica, R., Turiano, D., & Hammer, K. (2017). The fascinating history of bergamot (citrus bergamia risso & poiteau), the exclusive essence of Calabria: A Review. *Journal of Environmental Science and Engineering A, 6*(1). https://doi.org/10.17265/2162-5298/2017.01.003

McCracken, M. (n.d.). Goldenseal, Hydrastis Canadensis L.: A Long And Colorful Folk History Native Plant. https://www.mastergardenersmecklenburg.org/goldenseal-hydrastis-canadensis-l-a-long-and-colorful-folk-history-native-plant.html

Mount Sinai. (2021). *St. John's wort*. Mount Sinai Health System. https://www.mountsinai.org/health-library/herb/st-johns-wort

Perez, J. (2018). *Food as Medicine Buckwheat (Fagopyrum esculentum; F. tataricum, Polygonaceae)*. Food as medicinebuckwheat (Fagopyrum esculentum; F. Tataricum, Polygonaceae) - american botanical council. https://www.herbalgram.org/resources/herbalegram/volumes/volume-15/number-10-october/food-as-medicine-buckwheat

Petre, A. (2020, June 18). Goldenseal: Benefits, Dosage, Side Effects, and More. https://www.healthline.com/health/goldenseal-cure-for-everything

Pivarnik, P. B. M. (2019, October 14). *The history, mythology, and offerings of Hawthorn*. Herbal Academy. https://theherbalacademy.com/hawthorn-offerings/

Plant fact sheet - USDA. USDA -Natural Resources Conservation Services. (2017). https://plants.usda.gov/DocumentLibrary/factsheet/doc/fs_glle3.docx

Raman, R. (2018, October 25). Echinacea: Benefits, Uses, Side Effects and Dosage. https://www.healthline.com/nutrition/echinacea#antioxidants

Raman, R. (2019, January 25). What Is Feverfew? Benefits, Migraine Impact, and More. https://www.healthline.com/nutrition/feverfew

Rivlin, R. (2001, March 03). Historical Perspective on the Use of Garlic, *The Journal of Nutrition*, Volume 131, Issue 3, March 2001, Pages 951S–954S, https://doi.org/10.1093/jn/131.3.951S

Shoemaker, S. (2020, October 01). Angelica Root: Benefits, Uses, and Side Effects. https://www.healthline.com/nutrition/angelica-root#uses

WebMD. (2018). *Ginkgo: Overview, uses, side effects, precautions, interactions, dosing and reviews*. WebMD. https://www.webmd.com/vitamins/ai/ingredientmono-333/ginkgo

Zielinski, E. (2021, January 11). 9 Benefits Of Bergamot Essential Oil: Anxiety, Pain & More! https://naturallivingfamily.com/9-benefits-of-bergamot-essential-oil

Vogel, A. (2021). *Salvia officinalis L.* Salvia officinalis L. | Sage | Plant Encyclopedia | A.Vogel. https://www.avogel.com/plant-encyclopaedia/salvia_officinalis.php

Chapter 7

Carter, M., & Mckyes, E. (2005). Cultivation And Tillage. *Encyclopedia of Soils in the Environment*, 356-361. http://doi:10.1016/b0-12-348530-4/00514-2

Codekas, C. (2016, August 05). 6 tips for storing dried herbs. https://theherbalacademy.com/6-tips-for-storing-dried-herbs/

Jabbour, N. (2021, June 18). How to harvest herbs: How and when to harvest homegrown herbs. https://savvygardening.com/how-to-harvest-herbs/

McVicar, J. (2010). *Grow Herbs: An Inspiring Guide to Growing and Using Herbs*. Penguin.

Rana, S. (2017, December 05). The right way to store fresh and dried herbs: Expert tips. https://food.ndtv.com/food-drinks/the-right-way-to-store-fresh-and-dried-herbs-expert-tips-1783908

Chapter 8

Bridget, A, Z., Maslowski, D., Johnson, C., Langlois, C., B, L., . . . Cassandra. (2021, February 25). Learn How To Make Your Own DIY Essential Oils. https://www.diynatural.com/diy-essential-oils/

Herbal healing cream. (n.d.). https://www.herbalremediesadvice.org/herbal-healing-cream.html

Colgate. n.d. Making a Natural Mouthwash Recipe with Essential Oils. https://www.colgate.com/en-us/oral-health/selecting-dental-products/making-a-natural-mouthwash-recipe-with-essential-oils

Kendle. (2018, September 14). How to Make Herbal Infusions & Decoctions for Wellness Support. https://blog.mountainroseherbs.com/herbal-infusions-and-decoctions

Santos-Longhurst, A. (2019, May 17). Poultice: How to Make Your Own Herbal Anti-Inflammatory Paste. https://www.healthline.com/health/poultice

Chappell, S. (2019, December 18). A Beginner's Guide to Making Herbal Salves and Lotions. https://www.healthline.com/health/diy-herbal-salves#types

Dessinger, H. (2021, October 20). 16 Types of Herbal Remedies & How To Make Them (Tinctures, Elixirs, Decoctions, & More). https://mommypotamus.com/types-of-herbal-remedies/

Chapter 9

Chevallier, A. 2016. *Encyclopedia of herbal medicine* (3rd ed). DK.

Printed in Great Britain
by Amazon